Peculiar Beauty

Peculiar Beauty

Three Centuries of

Charmingly Absurd Advice

Bonnie Downing

Carroll & Graf Publishers
New York

PECULIAR BEAUTY

Carroll & Graf Publishers
An Imprint of Avalon Publishing Group Inc.
245 West 17th Street
New York, NY 10011

AVALON
publishing group incorporated

Library of Congress Cataloging-in-Publication Data is available.

ISBN: 0-7867-1450-6

Printed in the United States of America
Interior design by Simon Sullivan and Maria Elias
Distributed by Publishers Group West

For Molly FitzSimons and for my sister, Laura.

Contents

Peculiar Beauty

Introduction

My obsession started in third grade, in my best friend's basement. Her mother, a Mary Kay lady, had turned the recroom into a beauty lab. The makeup was fun, and I was intrigued by a curious display designed to prove some point about face creams. The setup involved three prunes, each in a baby food jar. One floated in oil, one stayed plump submerged in water, and the third was dry and shriveled. But my favorite thing in that basement was the book revered as a bible, that eighties classic *Color Me Beautiful,* by Carole Jackson. I never managed to determine what "season" I was, but beauty manuals have been my guilty pleasure ever since.

I hunt them down at every stoop sale, every trip to used book stores, and at every library I visit. When I realized last year that I have the Dewey Decimal number for *"beauty, personal"* memorized, I decided to do this book.

The outlandish tips amuse me, but the books also soothe me. They combine the charm and glamor of an old movie and the whole-new-you fun of leafing through fashion magazines.

Collected here are the most bizarre bits of advice from this underappreciated genre, dating from the late 1700s up to today. You'll hear from world-famous celebrities, beauty icons, and housewives who wrote books based on formulas passed down from their grandmothers. I hope you'll laugh out loud when you read suggestions to wash your hair in gasoline, or to add spinach leaves to the bath—but really, is any of it stranger than Botox?

As sweetly outdated and amusing as much of the advice can be, I can't help but notice that most of our thoughts on beauty have come full circle. Low-carb diets seem like the newest craze, but diets recommended for weight loss dating as far back as the early 1800s were all based on small servings of lean meat or fish and vegetables. Today's Pilates classes are based on movements found in calisthenic routines throughout modern history. What we now call alpha-hydroxy acid treatments have always been around—in the form of milk baths and lemon juice facials.

I love the do-it-yourself spirit of these authors. Predictably, many of these books were written by celebrities consumed by their appearances. It's humanizing to think of a time when, instead of an actress scheduling a personal trainer or running off for liposuction, she worked out at a home gym comprised of a chair, a broomstick, and a box of salt.

Many of my authors started their own beauty companies. In fact, during the course of my research, I found a bunch on the home shopping channels, selling new lines of beauty products.

There are a few male gurus featured here: Benjamin Gayelord Hauser, Way Bandy, and George Masters were all icons of their times. But most of the quotes in this book are by women. The beauty business has long been a popular way for women to enter the workforce. Like cooking, it was a way to make money by instinct—to use the knowledge they grew up with, and the skills they exhibit every day.

C. J. Walker, this country's first black female millionaire, made her fortune with a homemade hair tonic. Last year, when the Kabul Beauty School was opened in war-torn Afghanistan, the graduating students became among the highest female earners in their country. Their training (and new looks!) brought them restored confidence and an opportunity for self-expression after years behind burkas.

Self-expression is the essence of the beauty guide. In choosing quotes, I look for voice, narrative, mini-stories. The books are so personal, so confessional. These are auto-beauty-ographies: They are intended as how-to guides, but they emerge as personal diaries and cultural artifacts.

This book continues a long and intimate conversation between women. You will really get to know all the authors in their most private moments, perched on bathroom counters, slathering themselves with homemade potions, sometimes giggling and sometimes dead serious. But always, always trying to look their best.

Bonnie Downing
Brooklyn
June 17, 2004

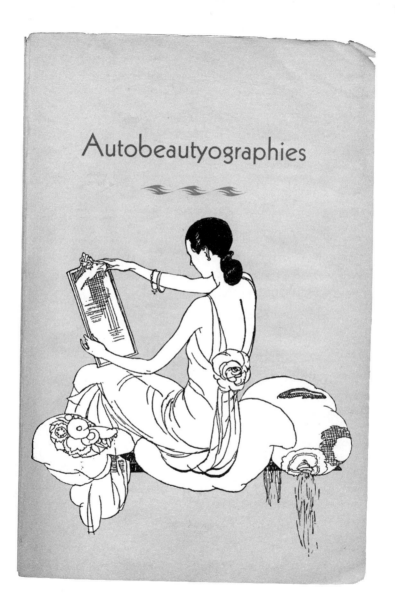

Autobeautyographies

~≋~

Party beauty from Andy Warhol's entourage, extreme sibling relationships, and why finding a husband is just like shopping. This is a chapter of exhibitionists, but you'll also hear from people who reveal way more about their lives than they intended, or simply paint an unforgettable picture. Autobeautyographies are a genre of their own: beauty manuals as real-life stories.

~≋~

I adore artifice. I always have. I remember when I was thirteen or fourteen buying red lacquer in Chinatown for my fingernails. . . . So I went around with these red red fingernails—you can imagine how that would have gone over at the Brearley School.

Then . . . when I started going out a few years later, I discovered calcimine. If I was going out— and I went out almost every night—two and a half hours before my escort arrived I'd start with this huge bottle of calcimine—a sponge . . . and I'd be totally calcimined from the waist up, out along the arms, the throat, et cetera, et cetera. I had to do this alone, because my family didn't take much interest in what I was doing. Then, when my escort and I would get up to dance, he, in his black dinner jacket, would be totally white. I would come off on him. But he'd have to put up with it. It meant nothing to me—I looked like a lily!

~Diana Vreeland,
DV (1984)

First of all, let me say that every girl can be attractive.
   "Oh," you say, "it's easy for you to talk, you're a model."
Of course, you are right. I am a model.

~Betty Cornell,
Betty Cornell's Teen-Age Popularity Guide (1953)

Certainly, without a sense of humor I would never have used one of my most effective diet tricks. Someone told me that Debbie Reynolds kept a photograph of me taken during my fattest period on her refrigerator door. She said it reminded her of what could happen if she charged into the icebox. During the initial stage of my diet I thought, well, if it works for Debbie, maybe it will work for me. I stuck a picture of myself at my worst on the refrigerator, and every time I went to the kitchen, there was my corpulent self reminding me of what would happen if I broke my diet. That sight was an excellent deterrent to binging. If you think a picture of me as Miss Lard will inspire you, go ahead and put it on your refrigerator, I have no objection. Certainly there are enough photos for you to choose from. I didn't exactly skulk about in those days, and even if I had tried to avoid the press, they would have found me.

~**Elizabeth Taylor,**
Elizabeth Takes Off (1987)

No sooner than you have decided to go on even a mild diet than you may feel sad. Many women are overwhelmed by a feeling that echoes from childhood. (No chocolate pudding for Jane tonight . . . because she stuck out her tongue at her cousin . . . because she forgot to feed poor Dickie bird his seed . . . because she simply will not pay attention.) The whole feeling is one of loss and deprivation. It's true that dieting does mean cutting out certain things. You won't be seeing any Baked Alaska for a while.

~The Editors of Harper's Bazaar,
Harper's Bazaar Book of Beauty (1959)

To a tub half full of water, add one pound of table salt and one pint of violet ammonia. . . . While in the tub I play about as joyfully as a young porpoise. I plunge and flounder and toss up a shower of water with my hands; for to lie lazily in a tub of water is to invite rheumatism and neuralgia.

~Lina Cavalieri,
My Secrets of Beauty (1914)

Most women complain that they cannot take cold baths—not because of ill health, but because the shock of the cold water is too much for them. I have a way of getting into my cold bath that overcomes this shock. This method always interests the women who attend my special matinees. They cannot understand why my feet go into the water last instead of first.

This is my system: I grasp the sides of the tub and lower my body into the water so that the base of my spine touches the water first. Then I lower the upper part of my body until the water touches the base of the brain, at the same time splashing my chest and throat. Then I let my feet down and I am wet all over.

~Edna Hopper Wallace,
My Secrets of Youth and Beauty (1925)

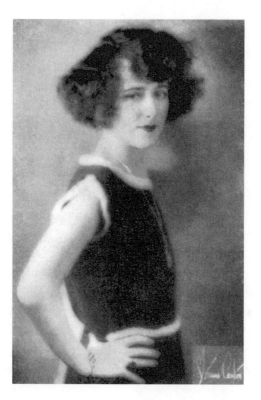

Edna Wallace Hopper was the original peculiar beauty. A huge star on Broadway and in silent films, she also had her own successful cosmetic company and modeled for all her own ads. She went on to have a popular radio show during which she further extolled the virtues of her potions. Perhaps most notable, though, are the matinees to which this ad refers. Edna had a stage set built to perfectly resemble her own bed and bathrooms, and only women were allowed to purchase tickets to see Edna perform her daily grooming and fitness rituals. Throughout her book, she makes readers aware that she has never personally experienced any of the beauty problems she writes about—never a blemish, and never more than "two pounds overweight."

Edna's methods worked so well, in fact, that as she tells us in her book, she once had to sign a legal document stating that she was indeed not her own granddaughter. The manager of a theater where she was working at the time needed proof to answer the complaints he received that Edna was a fraud. It seems her audiences were just that astounded by how young she looked.

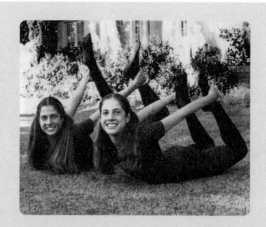

The Double-Energy Twins

Shari and Judi Zucker were seventeen years old when they co-authored **How to Survive Snack Attacks . . . Naturally.** The book of vegetarian recipes and exercise tips sold over half a million copies. The twins made appearances on television talk shows like Merv Griffin, and then became the **Nature Valley Granola** twins.

To say that Shari and Judi have remained close is a vast understatement. The twins live within a couple miles of each other and leave their houses every morning before dawn, mini-flashlights in hand, to meet halfway and go for a run together. "We never run out of things to talk about," says Shari. "Every day is like a holiday with my twin sister."

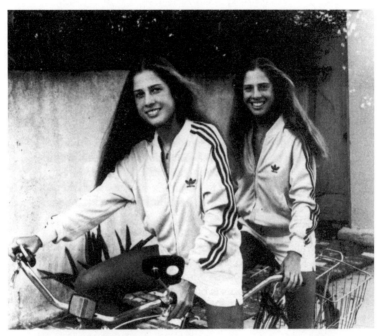

Bike riding is good exercise for almost everyone. We do it in double time on our bicycle built for two.

No lady ever leaves a ring in the tub. It's a disgusting sight for the next person who may have to use that bathroom and it's a bad example for children if there are any (there usually are, somewhere around). Make an exercise of cleaning the tub. Put a little extra touch of soap on your nail brush and twist around as far as you can, give a couple of quick swipes around that line which hard water and soap leave, and whisk it right out of sight. Just before you stand to your feet and let the water drain out. When you step out of the tub, you have combined a healthful practice of leaving a clean tub and twisting yourself at the same time.

~Margery Wilson,
You're As Young As You Act (1951)

I always try to avoid chemical cosmetics and seek out edible items to use on my skin and hair. Through the years, I've broken and scrambled dozens of eggs over my head for shampoo, added a dash of rum to camouflage the egg aroma, and squeezed on lemon juice as a natural rinse to achieve a high shine. Now I fill the sink with violets, run hot water over them, boil them, squeeze them, all but stamp on them, but to no avail. I cannot coax out of the petals a convincing violet tint. I make a foray to the greengrocer's and come home with samples of purple broccoli, dark red grapes, beets, cranberries, red plums—anything that has a red-purple hue. Then I experiment.

Cranberry juice or liquid cranberry jelly proves most satisfactory on my hair. It gives a vibrant red sheen to my dark brown hair, which I wear loose and wild. I wash it in the red juice, shake it out to dry, never let a comb near it, and glory in my snaky ringlets, untamed by human hands. Using fresh beets on my cheeks and lips, I achieve an alive transparent tint.

To renew my lip color during the evening I pull out of my gold mesh evening purse a gigantic fresh beet with the green leaves still dangling on their red stems. With a tiny gold knife I slice a morsel from the beet and rub it on my lips and cheeks in full view of the staring onlookers. The shade it imparts is neither red nor pink nor orange but an out-of-this-world rouge-violet. Try it sometime. I take the beet and the leaves home and eat them the next day. And more than once, when there is a long wait between meals, I head off starvation by nibbling a few mouthfuls of the white rice powder that I dust on my face from a beautiful cloisonné compact.

For my eyes, I forgo the natural approach and buy false lashes by the yard. I glue a four-inch strip on my upper and lower lids, letting it run all the way back to my hairline, as if the lashes were born out of my corkscrew hair. With my centipede eyes, I conquer hundreds of hearts. And on rainy days, when the dampness turns my Medusa locks into a huge ostrich feather duster, I enhance the effect by wearing white ostrich feathers in my hair.

~Ultra Violet,
Famous for 15 Minutes (1988)

Nature set us a tough task in understanding our complicated human mechanisms. But she furnished a key to her own mysteries by creating a color code of personality to read.

Pet Sins
Blondes:

1. Blondes repress their natural oomph by feeling inferior in social situations.
2. Blondes who have not learned to compensate properly may be fickle, frivolous, selfish, cold and gold-digging.

Brunettes:

1. Brown-eyed brunettes who place material values before love are likely to exploit friends or lovers for selfish purposes.
2. Brunettes have many secret fears and worries; they frequently worry themselves into a neurotic state.

Redheads:

1. Redheads show less compliance with things or submission to people than any other type; they have an extreme temperament if not temper.
2. Redheads are chronic kibitzers; they cannot keep out of other people's business, and they are apt to be calamity howlers.

~Babs Lee,
ABC's of Beauty (1950)

Marcia, Marcia, Marcia!
The Strange Case of Edith Carter
From Duckling to Swan is a nineteen-page pamphlet that tells the story of how Edith Carter used prayer and self hypnosis to surpass her sister's beauty. Look for more from Edith in the Magical Thinking chapter, and please note: When Edith started this quest she was in her mid-forties.

You can feel and look prettier, and years younger, by using these suggestions I have mentioned, and the things I'm going to tell you about.

Now, for the details of my change: Sister Mary was left a widow. As she had never had to support herself, I took her into business with me. It was the same old story. Compliments came to Mary all the time. People just couldn't realize we were sisters.

I could stand no more. I hastened to the restroom. Something seemed to go through me like electricity, so great was my wound and my determination. With all the force, vehemence and earnestness I seemed to possess, I put my foot down and declared, "I WILL BE PRETTY. PRETTIER THAN MY SISTER."

I didn't know just how I was going to do it. I only knew I was determined to do it. And the bible said, "Thou shall decree a thing and it shall be so unto thee." And remember, I was a matured woman.

~Edith Carter,
From Duckling to Swan (1948)

J'm Screaming Jnside

Learn to smile with your mouth closed. Work until you can do it in such a convincing manner that you are sure you're laughing with your mouth wide open.

~Wendy Ward,
Wendy Ward's Charm Book (1972)

To firm up the muscles that support the breasts (not the breasts themselves), smile as widely as you can (until it turns into a grimace), hold for a count of ten, and release. Repeat five times.

~Linda Stasi,
Looking Good Is the Best Revenge (1984)

We have all heard that physicians believe civilized people need to be well dressed and that they sometimes advise women who are ill mentally to go out and have a real "splurge" in buying dresses and hats.

~**Grace Margaret Morton,**
The Arts of Costume and Personal Appearance (1943)

Tweed knickerbockers are considered quite the thing abroad, to wear with tailor-made walking costumes — a very wise precaution indeed, for nothing can be more revolting to gaze upon than a white petticoat that has been worn on a muddy day, and no amount of care can prevent its bedraggled flounces from soiling the chaussure. A woman who wears knickerbockers and gaiters under her skirt for walking, comes home in a trim condition very pleasant to see, and the fatigue of holding up a train and several petticoats to keep them from dipping in the mud having spared to her, she is generally in a charming temper, a fact which enchants husbands and renders them great advocates of "the knickerbockers craze."

~**The Marquise de Fontenoy,**
Eve's Glossary (1897)

First the Morning Face. This is the face that the homemaker must show to her family. It should look fresh, unworried, and composed. Your whole

appearance must be as shining and as fresh as your
will power and determination can make it. It will
mean, perhaps, rising a bit earlier in the morning,
using a few precious minutes for quickly cleansing the
face, and applying a quick morning makeup. You can
then face your family and your day with new courage.
If there is no family you will have to face yourself.

~Edyth Thornton McLeod,
Lady, Be Lovely (1955)

To me a good way to shop is ask yourself two questions:
- Do I really need it?
- Do I really love it?

If you can answer "Yes" to both, go to it, baby!

The career or college girl who rushes into marriage
because everyone else is doing it often finds that
getting there is all the fun. Courtship, engagement, and
the flurry of plans for a wedding are a form of heady
stardom . . . even if you don't *exactly* know for sure
whether you want to add a hot stove to your already
humming electric typewriter.

The two questions become
- Do I really need him?
- Do I really love him?

~Eve Nelson,
Take It From Eve (1968)

Wear bikini pants or nothing and slather Andrea Extra
Strength Crème Bleach—a nice thick paste—over
thighs, calves, arms, your whole body if you like.
Leave on ten minutes and don't mess with it. Now
start rubbing with your hands . . . stroke stroke stroke
rub rub rub. Dead skin will come off with the dried
bleach—a most gratifying experience.

~Helen Gurley Brown,
The Late Show (1993)

Q. Do you analyze your looks?
A. What I do is just get in the shower with all my
make-up on and let it run all over my face. And when
the mascara smears and all the black starts smearing
over your cheeks, you just take all that off and look
incredible. Or take a shower and let the mirror frost up
and look at yourself that way, if you're really hopeless.

~Patti D'Arbanville being interviewed by **Francesco Scavullo**
in Scavullo On Beauty (1976)

For causing the eyebrows to grow when lost by fire, use
the sulphate of quinine—five grains in an ounce of alcohol.

~Mrs. Susan C. D. Power,
The Ugly-Girl Papers (1874)

Chew gum (in private, of course) with your head thrown back and your jaws working like mad.

~**Ruth Harper Larison,**
Those Enduring Young Charms (1942)

Q. How do you take care of yourself?
A. I take ballet and wrap my thighs in Saran Wrap: it's like another skin, and I lose water from any of the spots that are wrapped.

~**Mary Tyler Moore,**
being interviewed by **Francesco Scavullo** in Scavullo on Beauty (1976)

When I was a little girl, I was often reprimanded for admiring myself in the mirror. But I say to you, never lose an opportunity to look into every mirror you pass, but always do so from the corner of your eyes.

~**Madame Josephine Jaquet,**
I Wander and I Ponder (1936)

Overkill

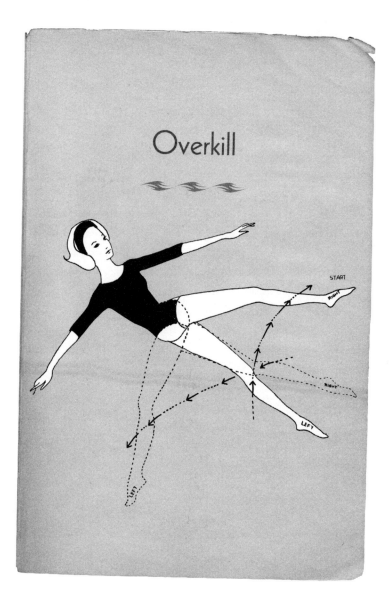

Why going feral is good for your nails, how old shoes and too much eye makeup can kill you, and what The Devil invented to keep you from slimness. Sometimes we all go too far. This chapter is the place for it—strong language and stronger opinions. Featuring enigmatic diagrams, wool bathing suits, and why broken nails are the Worst Thing Ever.

If a girl has the trial of a complexion so bad that the sight of it gives one a turn, it is simply a duty for her either to not go into society at all, or, if she does, to conceal it as she would not scruple to conceal lameness and leanness. You have no right to inflict your misfortune on everybody — it is an unpardonable offence against good taste.

~Mrs. H. R. Haweis,
The Art of Beauty (1878)

Women who have a tendency to a downy fuzz on their face should be very careful to remove all cold cream. Even though the cream may not cause hair to grow, it does make the down shiny and therefore more conspicuous.

~Edith Porter Lapish & Flora G. Orr,
Be Beautiful (1932)

One broken nail can make you look and feel sloppier than almost anything else. Most girls keep such a fingernail hidden whenever possible, for they appreciate the value of good-looking nails. Smooth, well-cared for fingertips convey an impression of smart spruceness. Hands are always in evidence — across a table, around a cocktail glass, at a bridge game, at a desk — and when well-groomed they mark a girl as up-to-date and fastidious. Of course, a girl may have sterling qualities and yet not have the good habit of caring for her nails, but neglect in this one detail may give other people the impression that she is slovenly and careless in everything.

~Mary MacFadyen, M.D.,
Beauty Plus (1938)

I believe one of the most important beauty habits that should be started early is a face-fix fund—for your nose bob, eye job, or anything else that needs fixing. Mothers should start this for their offspring in a child's piggy bank. Or in a special savings account at the bank in the child's name. Older children should be encouraged to save a certain amount of money regularly in their face-fix fund, just as they save each year in a Christmas Club fund. Young girls who start working as soon as they're out of school should start a face fund. If they start at eighteen or nineteen, saving fifty dollars a year in their face funds—the amount they usually save in their Christmas funds—they will have a good nest egg for a mini-tuck when they need it.

All women should have a face-fix fund, even if they have to sneak it out of the family budget, so that when the time comes for the snips and tucks they will be prepared.

~George Masters,
The Masters Way to Beauty (1977)

Too busy? Ah, there's the rub. The eternal question is: shall I go upstairs and pop a pimple or stay down here and cook papa's supper? I can't help you decide the ethical puzzle. For beauty you need time. Time is the most costly thing there is. Even the idlest matron, curled in the lap of luxury, knows something about the price of hours and minutes.

You may throw this book in the ash-can.

Because you may be after something more valuable than beauty.

If you have found anything answering that description, I'd like to hear about it. Give a girl a tip.

~Sylvia Ullback's secretary,
Hollywood Undressed, observations of Sylvia as noted by her secretary (1931)

Secretary? Or Alter-Ego?
Although I have also quoted from Sylvia Ullback's other books (all written in her distinctive voice), it is the enigmatic **Hollywood Undressed**, attributed to her secretary, that intrigues me the most.

Ms. Ullback is listed as the author of **Hollywood Undressed** inside the front cover, and the subtitle describes the book as Sylvia's observations. Yet it is all written from the perspective of a watchful, unnamed secretary. I am still unclear as to whether this was an amusing little alter-ego or a real person.

EYES: Open.

GENERAL RULE: Most of our lives are fraught with small or large stress situations, little and big problems—*and it is precisely these situations that play havoc with our facial control and accelerate our aging speed.* Therefore, by becoming mistress of your face in these situations, *you will also become mistress of your apparent age!* You must comprehend all of the situations *with a total lack* of facial movement. You will FEEL, be AWARE: *but your face will remain motionless. The sensitive placement of your hands and fingers will inform you of how quiet you can maintain your facial muscles.*

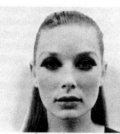

1. *Smile,* without motion (to the count of five). Do not move the corners of your mouth. 1-2-3-4-5.

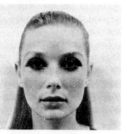

2. *Frown,* without moving your eyebrows or forehead (to the count of five). 1-2-3-4-5.

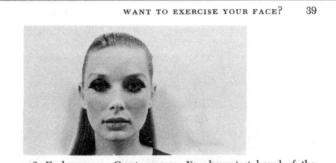

3. Feel *concern*: Great concern. You have just heard of the enormous financial loss suffered by your best friend (to the count of five). 1-2-3-4-5.

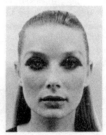

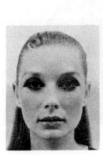

4. *Stress*: You are a half hour late for an appointment with your husband's employer. Without your husband's knowledge, you had arranged this meeting to request an increase in salary for him. You were to meet on a street corner, at a busy intersection, beneath a clock. You must get there at once! Feel stress without moving a muscle. 1-2-3-4-5.

5. *Pain*: You just stubbed your big toe against a rock. Feel pain without facial motion (to the count of five). 1-2-3-4-5.

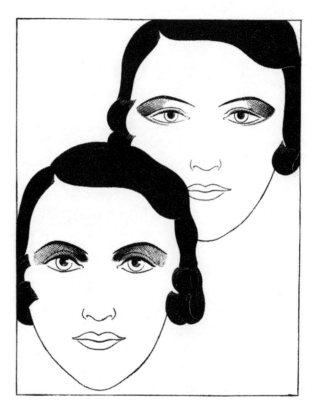

Study the next hundred women you see. Why do so many have pasty, muddy, blotched, or sallow skin? Why are there so many ungraceful double or triple chins? Why do so many women have a shapeless mass of sagging wrinkles instead of what should be that lovely part of the face — the firm, smooth curve from ear to chin?

~Belle Armstrong Whitney
What to Wear (1916)

I believe every woman — especially with today's eye makeup fashions — should keep a constant DANGER sign in her mind, before she blithely embarks on a program that may lead to facial disaster in a very few years.

I am referring to the blandishments of cosmetic manufacturers which invoke young girls (and their mothers) to a program of eye makeup, the constant use of which may have a demolishing effect on skin structure and firmness. It is this trend toward the so-called "Twiggy" look that may prove fatal.

~Jessica Krane,
How to Use Your Hands to Save Your Face (1969)

If it's a healthy, glowing look you're after, buy proper cream or liquid rouge—soft and easily spreadable impermanent tint in cream. The best shades are those muddy-salmon paste tones, not the sharp fuchsia tones that stand off the face shouting I'm Rouge.

~Graeme Hall,
Beauty for Girls Who Are Getting On (1970)

It is agreed that those who are lean should nourish themselves with plenty of air and water, shunning stimulants, tobacco smoke, coffee, tea, and excitement.

~Francis Mary Steele and **Elizabeth Livingston Steele Adams,**
Beauty of Form and Grace of Vesture (1892)

I am sure that if I did not watch my weight carefully I would soon be overweight . . . I have never been more than two pounds overweight. But that was a warning. I made sure that I did not go on gaining.

~Edna Wallace Hopper
My Secrets of Youth and Beauty (1925)

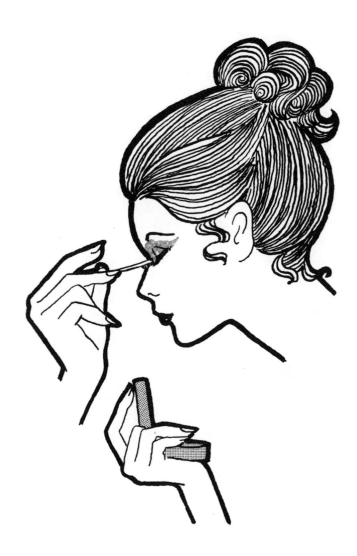

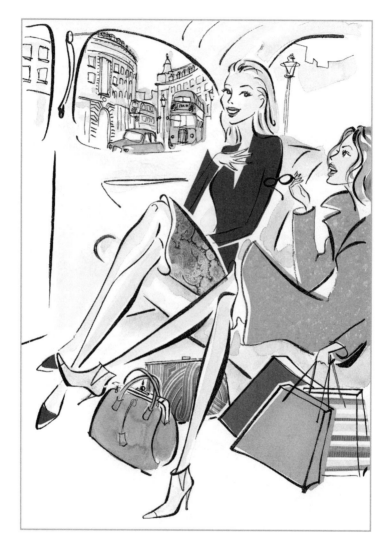

Make an emulsion of soft white soap, essence of turpentine, tincture of benzoin, essence of rosemary, and essence of Norwegian pine, in equal parts. Add two quarts thereof to the bath water, in which have been previously dissolved, four ounces of bi-carbonate of soda, a quart of spinach juice and twenty pounds of sea salt. This bath must be taken before going to bed and very hot.

~The Marquise de Fontenoy,
Eve's Glossary (1897)

At one time every lady of means possessed her still-room, where aromatic waters were distilled and various cosmetics compounded.

~Staney H. Redgrove,
The Cream of Beauty (1931)

It should not be forgotten that even when the teeth are pretty, white, and carefully attended to, the mouth cannot be called perfect unless the lips are in keeping with the rest. They should be of a fine ruby hue, soft, pliable, and, to use the favorite phrase of the novelists, "dewy." The vinegars and salves sold by perfumers and druggists to redden the lips are all humbug, if I may be permitted thus vigorously to express myself.

~The Marquise de Fontenoy,
Eve's Glossary (1897)

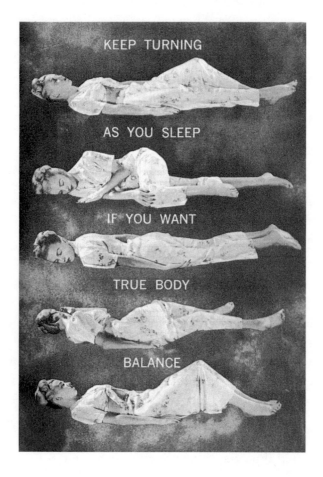

When Dr. Stillman recommended his eight glasses of water a day, it seemed to evoke groans from so many of his dieters. I couldn't understand it, since twenty glasses per day is the about the norm for me. (And yes—I know the location of every presentable ladies' room in the city of New York. But I don't have a pimple or a blown-up stomach.)

~MaryAnn Crenshaw,
The Natural Way to Super Beauty (1974)

Do not wear old shoes about the house. They will make your feet shapeless. The dyes in cheap stockings often run. If you have a slight skin abrasion or cut, you may get blood poisoning. Hence pay more for your stockings (silk, lisle or silk and wool) rather than risk infection.

~Florence Courtenay,
Physical Beauty (1922)

Is it in good taste for young girls to wear black? The problem is merely one of whether or not black is becoming. Black is the most unbecoming color in the world, by and large. It takes the life and vitality from the wearer. It is the color of death. It's much easier to wear black when you're young and vital then when you are old and gray. I would say that the only reason for not wearing black is that sometimes it depresses other people. To the extent to which you are concerned with the feelings of others, you might say it was good taste not to go about depressing them.

~Elizabeth Hawes,
Good Grooming (1942)

Perhaps Chanel's greatest gift to the working girl was her introduction of wool jersey to the fashion world. It looks good when made into casual clothes for the country, when made into sophisticated evening wear, and when made into spring coats (with suitable interlining), as well as for bathing suits and for hats.

~Bea Danville,
Dress Well on $1 a Day (1956)

In my school we teach our young beauty beginners to practice painting their lipline on paper. We use a plain sheet of typing or notebook paper. The girls bring into class an old, all but used-up tube of lipstick in a clear red shade. By working with your brush on paper, you quickly get used to the feel of the brush and the bristles. When a girl has extreme difficulty (in the

beginning) painting her lips on the paper, we give her
a lip pencil or a red china marker. Then, as she masters
her outline, we graduate her to a brush (on paper).

Because paper and skin have different surfaces,
before our young student starts outlining her lips, she
paints her lip imprint onto the inner surface of
her wrist.

~Candy Jones,
Time to Grow Up (1962)

Hypertrychosis, or Superfluous Hair.
This is one of the most annoying
and humiliating blemishes that
can befall the fair face of woman.
The writer personally knew of
one beautiful girl who
became so obsessed with
the dreadful fancy that
she was going to be
disfigured by superfluous
hairs that it unsettled her
mind and she committed
suicide.

~William A. Woodbury,
Beauty Culture (1910)

There is an old fashioned trick to help you discover what hairstyle is most appropriate and attractive for framing your face. First, apply foundation all over your face in an even and rather heavy coat (now is the only time I advocate clogging your pores like this, and it's only for a few minutes). The contrast between the base and your hair will help define your hairline. Then draw all of your hair back from your face, and secure it with a coated elastic or with clips. Stand about eight inches from a mirror and trace the outline of your face on the mirror with a piece of soap. Put a piece of tracing paper over the outline on the mirror and draw over it with a pencil. Then make several copies. Sketch in features—you don't need to be an artist, just approximate—and then experiment by drawing in different hairstyles.

~Evelyn Roaman,
The Evelyn Roaman Book (1981)

My friend's theory is that in evolution, what the body no longer has use for, it discards. When we were all living in the tree tops, swinging from branch to branch, and digging in the earth for food, nails were a useful implement necessary to survival. Today, we buy our potatoes washed, in polythene bags.

Nails, according to his theory, are on their way out;
and disintegration had already begun with this peeling

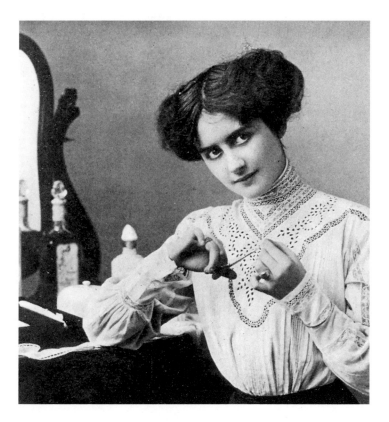

process in the next few hundred years, nails will be non-existent. I'm glad I shall not be around.

My nails were suffering at the time and he gave me a little experiment to try for myself.

"Every morning, scrape your nails on the trunk of a tree, really score the bark, if you can. Never mind if it tears them at first. They'll toughen up," he advised. His contribution was not exactly the advice I could incorporate in my weekly beauty column.

But he's right. Today, my nails are tough and long.

~Graeme Hall,
Beauty for Girls Who Are Getting On (1970)

The Devil could not be everywhere at once so he invented the frying pan!

~Benjamin Gayelord Hauser,
Mirror, Mirror on the Wall (1961)

Perhaps the Arab women, swathed in veils, and the Victorian maidens, screening their complexions with scarves and parasols, had the right idea. They knew that too much sun could turn skin into saddle leather. Luckily for me, my mother recognized this fact and insisted that I follow her example of wearing wide-brimmed sun hats during the summer months. Between us, we exceeded 50 — in all shapes, sizes, and colors. To this day, I have never acquired a sun tan!

~Arlene Dahl,
Always Ask a Man: Arlene Dahl's Key to Femininity (1965)

Nothing is more unfeminine than the straight line of the shoulder, which properly belongs to the cuirassier or an athlete. Some mothers make their young folks walk the floor with a pail of water in each hand, to give their shoulders a graceful droop. A substitute may be worn in one's room while at work, in the shape of an outside brace of triple gray linen, having two extra straps buckling round the tip of each shoulder, one long end reaching the belt, with a wedge-shaped lead or iron weight hooked on it. This is a heroic practice, but effectual; and its pains are amply compensated by lines of figure which are the surest exponents of high breeding.

~Mrs. Susan C. D. Power,
The Ugly-Girl Papers (1874)

Just how slippery are false eyelashes to handle?
You should know at once that, unless you're a first-time
lucky, the initial, cross-eyed, weepy application is utter
red-eyed hell. The lashes go everywhere but where you
want them. In your eyes, on the floor, and, unless
you've the patience to rip off the lot and start again, in
the bathroom waste-bin out of sheer frustration.
However, live through this baptism of tears, and you
would no more be seen at a party without your false
eyelashes that without your false teeth.

~Jean Rook,
Dressing for Success (1968)

Bad complexions cause more heartaches than crushed
ambitions and cases of sudden poverty. The reason is
plain. Ordinary troubles roll away from the mind of a
cheery, energetic woman like water from a duck's
back, but beauty worries—well! They have the most
amazingly insistent way of sticking to one. You may
say you won't think of them, but you do just the same.

~Mme. Qui Vive (Helen Follett Stevens),
The Woman Beautiful (1901)

That Certain Something

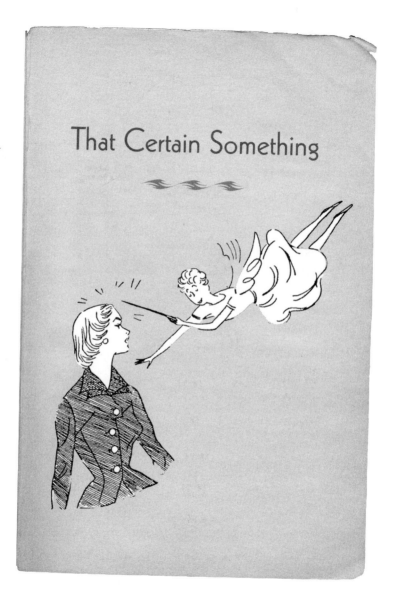

How to get in with the jitterbug crowd, what to hide in your décolleté, and what French women know that American women don't. Hear a brave voice fess up to the myriad forms of fulfillment that come only to the beautiful, and learn the importance of choosing a trademark mannerism.

Woman is most beautiful when she is most herself and least conscious of it.

~Mrs. H. R. Haweis,
The Art of Beauty (1878)

LET'S STUDY OUR GENERAL EFFECT, AS YOU ARE NOW. Arrange to study yourself before a large mirror. Is your walk that of a fat woman or a thin one? The effect is unmistakable.

One of my clients was a very thin woman, thin to the point of scrawniness. During the lesson I had her walk up and down the room while I studied her. Her walk puzzled me. I couldn't make it out. Finally it dawned on me that she walked as a fat woman walks. Slyly I said, "You have a fat friend, haven't you?" She stopped and turned a shining face to me. "Yes, did you see me with her?" She evidently loved and admired her friend very much. "No," I answered, "I didn't see you with her, but I see her with you right now. You have her walk, copied no doubt, unconsciously, because of your great affection for her." And so it goes with all of us.

WE HAVE ACQUIRED OUR MANNERISMS—WE MAY AS WELL ACQUIRE THE ONES WE WANT . . .

YOU WILL HAVE A TIMELESS PERSON-ALITY WHEN YOU HAVE RID YOURSELF OF

MANNERISMS, BOTH YOUTHFUL OR THOSE OF AGE. The youthful ones do not hurt, except that if you have mannerisms at all, they will gradually change with the years. So, the best thing to do is to rid yourself of mannerisms, then consciously choose one or two that would become your trademark and set you apart.

~Margery Wilson,
You're As Young As You Act (1951)

If you happen to be blessed with heavy, dry, and curly hair (think Gilda Radner) you can wear one of those gloriously frizzy halos that seem to go on forever. Cute.

~Gloria Richards,
A New You (1980)

Things happen to beautiful women. Things come to beautiful women. Material things, if you want them. Money and jewels and clothes and motors. Or things more real if you like. Friends, sympathy, contentment. People seek beauty. If you are beautiful, they will seek you, surround you, serve you. Love will come to you, a beautiful home, beautiful children. Fulfillment will come to you, meaning, a purpose in life.

There, I have dared to write them all down. These are

the reasons you want to be beautiful. Are they not? Why do we bother to evade and conceal them? They are the truth. And finer, more natural and significant truths than govern half our acts and longings . . . Beautiful women live fully, intensely, superbly. It has always been so.

~Dorothy Cocks,
The Etiquette of Beauty (1927)

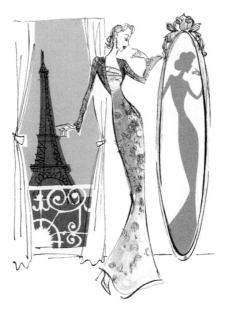

If you go night-clubbing, wear the deepest fuchsia-red lipstick you can find. It seems to glow in the half light. To add to your glamour you can sprinkle colored sequins in your hair after lightly spraying it with lacquer. You can brush them out the next day and be as prim as you please!

~**Edyth Thornton McLeod,**
Lady, Be Lovely (1955)

Those whose taste has been cultivated by having beautiful things always about them, are incredibly sensitive to awkward forms, inappropriate colours, and inharmonious combinations. To such persons, certain rooms, certain draperies, certain faces, cause not only the mere feeling of disapprobation, but even a kind of physical pain. Sometimes they might be unable to explain what affected them so unpleasantly, or how they were affected, but they feel an uneasy sense of oppression and discomfort—they would fain flee away, and let the simple skies or the moon with her sweet stare, soothe them into healthy feeling again.

~**Mrs. H. R. Haweis,**
The Art of Beauty (1878)

You know the rewards of beauty. You want to be admired and loved. You want to be the center of admiration in your own set. Then be it! Be loved and wanted and envied. *Be what you want to be!* Make yourself into the sort

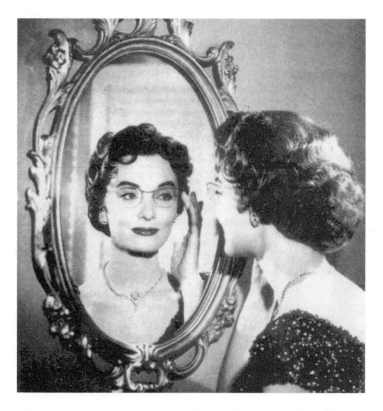

of woman you were meant to be; study yourself, and be
determined to make the most of what you possess. But
first of all, remember that no matter what your features or
the color of your hair may be; no matter how your
character may shine through your eyes or your teeth may
gleam; no matter how much Sex-Appeal you think you

have, you haven't got "IT"; you haven't found real beauty if you are not *in proportion.*

~Lilyan Malmstead,
What Everybody Wants to Know (1928)

If you're nice to be around, people generally want to have you around. That means you're popular; the longing to be popular is one of the keenest desires of the human heart.

~Seventeen's Beauty Workshop (1965)

I take a cotton ball and spray it with my favorite cologne. I plunge it into my cleavage. Some people call it décolleté. By whatever name it is called, it is a marvelous cachepot (hideaway) for scented cotton — terrific!

~Stella Reichman,
Great Big Beautiful Doll (1976)

Take my tip, girl, hold your tongue between your teeth. Every woman should have one secret about her appearance.

And one vanity. I have never been able to see why vanity should have been counted amongst the

Deadlies. It seems such a pathetic little sin. Every woman who is whole-hogging about her vanity seems to be committing a rather pallid evil: she's such a bore anyway that she has to sin alone because no one will stick her for long, poor dear!

~Graeme Hall,
Beauty for Girls Who Are Getting On (1970)

You must be vibrant. You must be alive, active, creative in your own life, able to meet every emergency with resilience. You must be all these things to be called youthfully beautiful in these modern times. Rhythmic speed and elastic poses are the symbols of the modern woman. The satin boudoir and the lady-like "vapors" of Victorian days are no longer fashionable.

~Helena Rubinstein,
Food for Beauty (1938)

Colorful speech does not imply talk which is filled with the latest words and phrases of the "jitterbug crowd." Occasionally, however, if one of these words is so comprehensive in its meaning that it fits your point to a "T," then use it! It shows your awareness of such things; that you are "on the beam." The very infrequency of slang in your conversation serves to accent its use when you do employ it, and consequently makes your remark more amusing.

~Veronica Dengel,
All About You (1953)

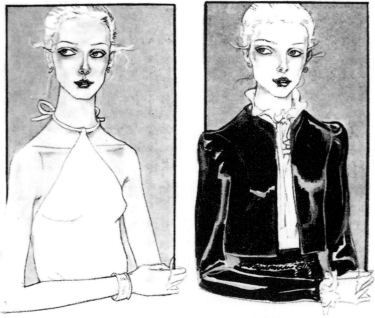

Wrong   Right

A French woman wears a fifty dollar dress and a fifteen dollar corset. An American woman wears a two hundred dollar dress and a two dollar and a-half corset.

~Amy Ayer,
Facts for Ladies (1908)

This brings me to another fashion. While it could hardly be called an American classic, it is showing all the signs of becoming a mainstay of many of our smartly dressed women. This is the caftan. The style we see most frequently originated in Morocco, and it's a natural for the older woman, whether she is as thin as Gloria Guinness or as well endowed as TV's Maude. One can't go to work in a caftan, but for entertaining at home, dining out or at resorts it's unbeatable. A caftan is almost as flexible as a dress, in that it can be as simple or as formal as you want. The lines, the shape of the garment is where the enormously feminine flattery lies. While every age group has adopted them, to the older woman they are a godsend. In a caftan, one is well covered but still very soft, very feminine-looking, with a hint of mystery that is attractive to men. I love the flow of the caftan as well as the great range of fabrics and styles.

~Pablo Manzoni,
Instant Beauty (1978)

Accessories are wonderful. I love them. And the best part is that they can be CHEAP, CHEAP, CHEAP, and no will ever know.

~Linda Stasi,
Looking Good is the Best Revenge (1984)

Take that $5 bill in your hand, go to the most reputable store in town, walk directly to the hat of your choice and declare your love. Let your instinct tell you what to do. If the hat fulfills your dream, buy it. Be strong, be firm, and don't ask anyone's advice. Don't try to make the hat look good on all your children and your friends, don't ask any questions — just buy. All great things are done impulsively. Sometimes they turn out to be the best choice you have ever made. If you do make a mistake, you learn from your mistake. The only real mistake is to take the problem too seriously. Go trust your subconscious integrity, don't waver, defy all gravity, let the $5 ride wherever it wants to go — it will be the best experience for $5 you have ever had.

~Mr. John,
The Charming Woman, edited by Helen Fraser (1950)

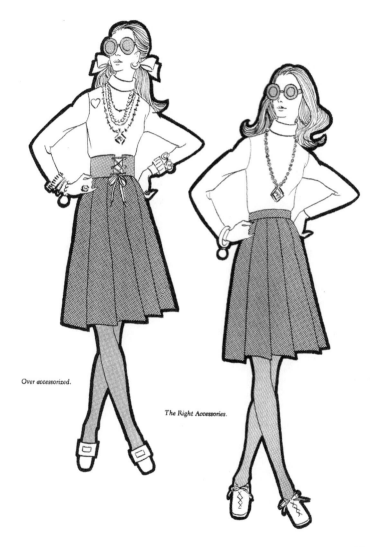

Over accessorized.

The Right Accessories.

At heart, every woman is a blonde. We've all dreamed of doing a Marilyn Monroe overnight. In fact, I truly believe that the only fulfilled woman is the one who had gone blonde once, if only for 12 hours.

~Jean Rook,
Dressing for Success (1968)

In short, a beauty is simply a girl who couldn't care more.

~Stan Place,
Stan Place's Guide to Makeup (1981)

The Ugly Truth

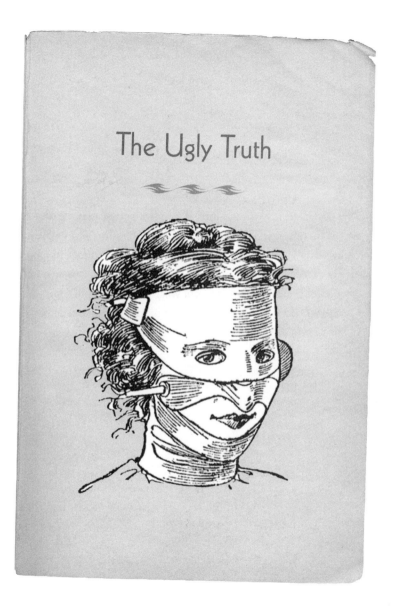

What America will always look at askance, several reasons why it would be best if you'd just shut up, and theories on why everyone is avoiding you: Is it your personality, or just body odor? I found nearly as many rants on ugliness as tips on loveliness. So, here is a chapter of brutal honesty. Find out what you're doing that just isn't working, and what to hide from your husband and confidantes.

American tastes, and morals too, will have to change entirely before smudged eyelids will ever be looked at in real life other than askance. The most lenient criticism it is possible to pass is that it gives a woman a doubtful appearance.

~**Ella Adelia Fletcher,**
The Woman Beautiful (1901)

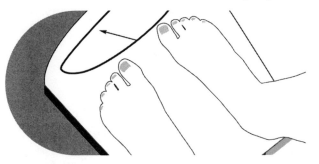

A great number of overweight women and men have really sold themselves the idea that they are persecuted by Nature in that everything they eat turns to fat. Their friends have given them sympathy over this sad plight.

But the fact in case is that such fat people during the war in countries where food was not available to satisfy their appetites, rapidly lost weight. Unless there is a definite glandular disturbance, which happens only in one out of a hundred thousand cases of overweight, the fat in the body is in ratio to the food intake and there is no other way about it.

THERE ARE NO OVERWEIGHT PEOPLE IN PRISON CAMPS.

~Margery Wilson,
You're As Young As You Act (1951)

It is the *duty* of woman to herself and to those who look upon her, to devote some part of every day, if only a few minutes, to the attainment and preservation of beauty, or the eradication of the many defacements of it.

~Elizabeth Hubbard,
Beauty, How Acquired and Retained (1910)

Every woman looks well in anything if you give her shadows enough. Beware of a brimless hat unless you are a great beauty, because it does not cast any shadows. Instead, it throws your complexion into relentless high 'relief' that is not flattering

~Belle Armstrong Whitney
What to Wear (1916)

Many women wish to improve their looks, but do not know how. Others fear that it may not be quite modest to make the effort.

~Belle Armstrong Whitney
What to Wear (1916)

Old fashioned people may protest and bewail the modern preoccupation in the cultivation of beauty as a manifestation of the laxness of the times. But I shall continue to regard it as a duty, and a virtue, as well as a distinct pleasure.

~Helena Rubinstein,
The Art of Feminine Beauty (1930)

One of our prominent Hollywood designers said recently in a public lecture on the subject of personal appearance, "Today if you are not beautiful you are truly dumb."

~Grace Margaret Morton,
The Arts of Costume and Personal Appearance (1943)

The phrase "attractively ugly" is not an empty one. An attractively ugly woman is one who knows how to create a pleasing whole out of ill-matched material. How could she do this if she did not first make a true estimate of her appearance?

~Jacqueline Du Pasquier,
A Guide to Elegance (1956)

You don't quite understand yourself. One day you're pleased with yourself. The next day you'd give your eye tooth to be someone entirely different. One day you're right in the swing of things and the next, for no good reason you can think of, you're overlooked completely. Your grades are good and you're just as attractive as the next girl. All these things are in your favor, but there's something wrong. What is it? Well, it could be your personality.

~Elsie Archer,
A Guide to Good Grooming for Negro Girls (1959)

Talking too much, idle chatter, can become such a waste of life. At times we are all guilty of it, from the housewife who chatters all day and leaves her dishes piled high in her electric kitchen, to the head salesman who can tell endless corny stories. If only we could learn to be silent unless we have something constructive to say, it would be a much more relaxed world to live in, and if ladies with loose tongues would remember to gossip less they would have fewer wrinkles around their mouths.

~Benjamin Gayelord Hauser,
Mirror, Mirror on the Wall (1961)

Avoid obscenity. . . . With rare exception, an obscene word is nothing more than a crude substitute for a better word. However, as with lying, there are some people who can get away with obscenity by employing it on the grand scale.

~**Quentin Crisp** and **Donald Carroll,**
Doing It With Style (1981)

And do remember that cosmetic preparations, however fine, cannot close the pores. The pores close only after you die!

~**Edyth Thornton McLeod,**
Lady, Be Lovely (1955)

White lashes and eyebrows are so disagreeably suggestive that one cannot blame their possessor for disguising them by a harmless device. A decoction of walnut-juice should be made in the season, and kept in a bottle for use the year round. It is to be applied with a small hair pencil to the brows and lashes, turning them to a rich brown, which harmonizes with fair hair.

~**Mrs. Susan C. D. Power,**
The Ugly-Girl Papers (1874)

Treat your hair kindly. Whether you wear it short or long, it is the frame and setting of your face. Even if you dislike the colour, never attempt to change it basically. There is always a subtle harmony of tone between your hair and your eyes, your skin and your temperament. Be very prudent in choosing and using dyes and bleaches. The radiance of a sallow skin surrounded by dark hair can be completely ruined by the substitution of a blond wig.

Above all, do not chop and change, from fair to red and red to dark. Nothing is more inelegant than experiments of that kind which justifiably annoy one's friends and acquaintances.

~Jacqueline Du Pasquier,
A Guide to Elegance (1954)

If you live a secluded life, among unsophisticated people, you should use very little make-up; otherwise, you will be out of place. But if you lead a social life, in Paris or London, colour your lips freely, or you will make a bad impression. When a woman is the only one in a group without make-up, she looks singularly unattractive — like a dim lamp beside a glittering chandelier.

~Jacqueline Du Pasquier,
A Guide to Elegance (1954)

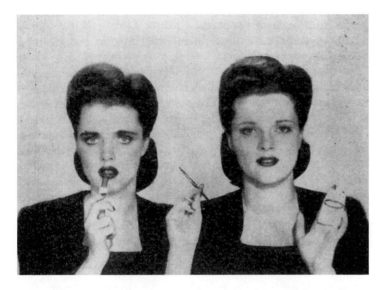

One day a week—Sunday in my case—I believe in resting the skin. No foundation cream, no powder, but always eyeliner and mascara. Unless you don't mind looking like a boiled egg.

~Jean Rook,
Dressing for Success (1968)

Don't forget how important the right "framing" of your large face is: many of us have short necks. Don't let your hair lie on your neck, it's ugly. Cut it short or put it up. Keep your neck uncluttered.

~Stella Reichman,
Great Big Beautiful Doll (1976)

To make a perfect job of back beautifying, determine first whether you are "Blimpy" or "Bumpy."

If you are "Blimpy", it means that disfiguring rolls of fat are obstructing the natural contour lines . . . bulging out from behind brassiere straps and over the top of your girdle. Your effort must be to reduce and to bring back firm, solid flesh.

If you are "Bumpy," your protruding ribs will make your back look like a xylophone. In this case, exercise and figure molding will tend to level off the back lines with a proper padding of muscle tissue.

~Joe Bonomo,
Reduce and Beautify Your Figure (1954)

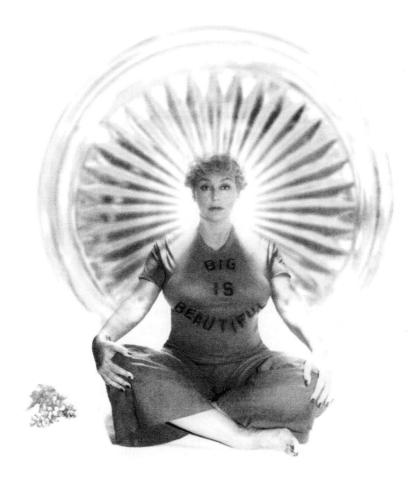

If you have been ten pounds overweight for the past ten years, you are officially obese. How do you like that word obese? Doesn't that rock you? The dictionary definition for obese is "extremely fat," from the Latin word "obesus" meaning "grown fat from eating." It may not seem that ten extra pounds is worth the categorizing as "extremely fat," but, as you may have found out, ten pounds and you keep on and on.

~Dorothy Seiffert,
Beauty for the Mature Woman (1977)

Keep your feet warm. Give those pretty round yellow silk garters to the girl you hate, and invest in sensible hose supporters. If your circulation is defective, wear wool stockings.

~Mme. Qui Vive (Helen Follett Stevens),
The Woman Beautiful (1901)

Of the habit of close observation that unfolds the truth with regard to what is becoming to us as individuals, we have precious little. It is not that we cannot learn, but that we will not. "What a pretty blouse," I say to a friend, and add with brutal frankness, "but you ought not to wear yellow."

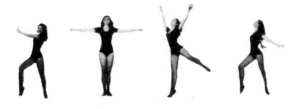

"Pshaw," says she, "what's the difference? I like yellow." And off she goes looking sallow and dull, and everybody who sees her and chances to have an "eye for color" shudders at her bad judgment.

~Belle Armstrong Whitney,
What to Wear (1916)

A buxom lass in overalls, with a mannish haircut, rolling a cigarette and handling sacks of fertilizer may be scrupulously scrubbed and as clean as a freshly bathed infant. But is she dainty? Is she "feminine"? Definitely not. . . . And while on this subject, let me remind some of you that ultra-smart, mannish suits and hats, plus "slicked back" hairdos, may make other women think you are the last word in fashion. But the man in your life—or the man you would like in your life—would much prefer you in something soft and clinging, preferably in color with dainty touches of white or other light colors here and there—and with your hair soft and fluffy around your face.

~LeLord Kordel,
Lady, Be Loved! (1953)

Never buy fabric gloves that pretend to be leather, for all forms of hypocrisy are poles away from elegance.

~Jacqueline Du Pasquier,
A Guide to Elegance (1956)

A stout woman cannot hope to achieve an attractive line. What she must do is to distract attention from her shape by neatness and fastidious attention to detail. Her appearance must be, in short, "exactly right." For this is her only way of being elegant. It may be true that a thoroughly well-proportioned, slim woman can allow herself to be careless on occasion without ruining her appearance; but for the larger woman, a crumpled skirt, a grubby blouse, or wispy hair inevitably makes her look like a slut.

~Jacqueline Du Pasquier,
A Guide to Elegance (1956)

You should never wear anything that pretends to be something it isn't: polyester pretending to be cotton, plastic pretending to be leather, and so forth. To do so is to fall victim to the Margarine Fallacy, which is the curious notion that something is valuable only insofar as it resembles something else. Thus, margarine is promoted on the basis of its resemblance to butter, synthetic materials are often judged by how convincingly they imitate "the real thing." In fact, they should be judged exactly as people should be judged—by how convincingly they imitate themselves. And, of course, by how convincingly they represent *you*.

> ~**Quentin Crisp** and **Donald Carroll**,
> Doing It With Style (1981)

It just might remain a mystery to you why you get left out of everything nice. If your best friend wouldn't tell you, *I* would. And supposing we worked or studied together, I'd start by asking you to tell *me* if I ever smelt even slightly stale or unpleasant, *because I know* that it's possible to get a little careless, or perhaps to use an anti-perspirant-deodorant that isn't effective for some reason (maybe it's time to change to a new one). I would talk in exaggerated terms about my absolute *horror* at the mere thought that I might smell of perspiration. And I would be putting on this act for your sake hoping that you would get the message.

~Mary Young,
The Best of Yourself (1970)

Look—Cheekbones!

Although I have found references to some form of facial contouring dating as far back as the twenties, the practice really became popular in the eighties. It was to faces what shoulder pads were to outfits—fierce, frightening, and overdone.

Of absolutely no help is the old trick of trying to hide full cheeks by means of cosmetic shading. It simply doesn't work. It's fine for a model who is professionally acquainted with her face and can color and shade it for the best camera and lighting advantages. But it won't do in real life. You cannot control the lights you're under or the angle at which people will look at you, nor can you remain in one position without moving your head. And every time any one of these three ordinary factors shifts just slightly, all of the shading you may have done is seen for just what it is — stripes of color on your face. I don't give any instructions for such application in this book, and if you should find it elsewhere, my advice is to ignore it. It has nothing to do with the real world. *Anything that shows what you've tried to do doubly defeats its own purpose.*

~Pablo Manzoni,
Instant Beauty (1978)

Just because chorus girls *have* to shave their legs and underarms, is no reason why women in general should turn up their nose at the practice. No young girl or matron wishes to appear in bathing costume with a generous covering of dark hair on her bare legs. Shave your legs, for here the razor gives the best results! Soaking the legs in warm water, and then rubbing them with pumice stone is a long process. It may "discourage" the hair, but then the hair may take years before it becomes properly discouraged.

~Florence Courtnenay,
Physical Beauty (1922)

The clever woman, who is also a loving and loyal wife, does not permit even her husband to cross the threshold of her dressing room while engaged in the mysteries of her toilet. Not that she has anything criminal to conceal, but because one can never escape from the fatal realisms of the toilet, however beautiful, poetical, graceful one may be. For example—a woman crimping her hair does not appear to advantage, and may even appear ridiculous. Besides, the trivialities of life always cause us to lose some of our prestige in the eyes of those who love us most. Therefore, let us not obtrude the prosaic thing of life on the attention of those who we most desire to please. It is unnecessary to remind the wise of our sex that, though in certain hours we may be goddesses, at other times we are only like all other women.

~Harriet Hubbard Ayer,
My Lady's Dressing Room (1892)

In the past, women had to act as if they had no excretory functions whatsoever. They sat and smiled, even though suffering acute discomfort, rather than run the risk of having anyone suspect they possessed any such function. They had to wait until an opportunity presented itself, no matter what the cost. And in those days it must have been very hard to sneak out, for there were no convenient bathrooms. Girls had to go in twos or more to an outhouse some distance away, and rain and cold and darkness were added hazards.

Today girls still maintain subterfuges, although a far more sensible attitude is taken. Thank goodness, however, that rest rooms and bathrooms are always unobtrusively handy. After a movie, for instance, it is

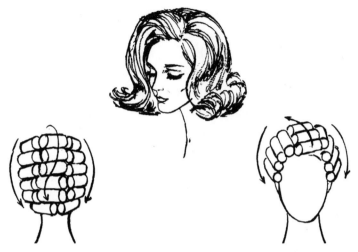

very easy for a girl to excuse herself without a blush, to "fix her hair," even though her curls obviously need no attention. The modern maiden knows she is fooling no one, and what does it matter anyway? Of course, one should avoid indecencies, but there is no need to suffer.

~Mary MacFadyen, M.D.,
Beauty Plus (1938)

Mentally remove your facial skin and look at the **skeletal structure** of your face and head. Where do the bones protrude? Where do the bones indent? Where are the valleys and mountains of your personal facial landscape?

Now get acquainted with your skin. Where is your skin fleshy? Loose? Tight? Close to the bone? Porous? Rough? Smooth? This kind of brutal analysis is necessary in order to know where and how you need to improve your appearance cosmetically. . . .
Now, if you haven't taken to your bed in despair, go for a walk and take a look at the faces of others. Ask the same questions—what a revelation!

~Way Bandy,
Designing Your Face (1977)

If women were allowed to wear out what they bought last season it would be impossible to sell them all new goods this, and the dividends on investments would be cut down or cut out. Therefore, men change the styles each season to force the sales of new clothes. Women lend themselves to this commercial whirligig. Whether they ought to or not is not the question—they do.

Theoretically, every woman ought to find the one style she looks best in, that she can afford to have, and always wear this style of garment. But in practice this is as far off as the millennium.

~Belle Armstrong Whitney,
What to Wear (1916)

Hairstyles for Zombies?

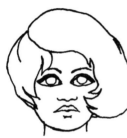

Round

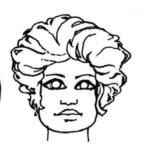

Pear

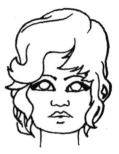

Square

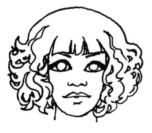

Long

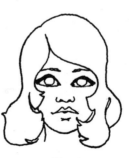

Heart

However you accent with rouge, do so lightly. Apply very little rouge in the morning, when your cheeks are inclined to be pale. Later, when activity brings a natural blush to your face, you can add a little more if you still need it.

But remember the pathetic statement, "Too much rouge is a sign of despair."

~Arlene Dahl,
Always Ask a Man: Arlene Dahl's Key to Femininity (1965)

Magical Thinking

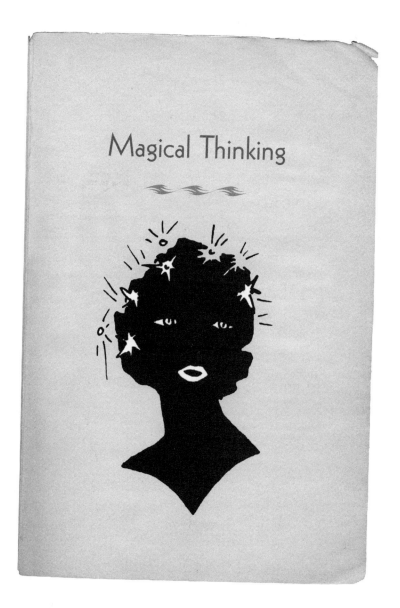

Self-hypnosis, supernatural potions, and finding Jesus. Find out whether wishing really will make it so, and why you owe it to your Creator to work out. Plus unusual interpretations of the Bible, what good clothes can do that religion never could, and visits from both the patron saint of lost causes and Satan himself.

Place in your sleeping chamber a likeness picture of how you would like to look (naturally using common sense), and morning and night, and at any convenient time during the day when you come before that picture say soulfully and earnestly, *The perfect mind within me is refashioning and reconstructing my features in accordance with that image.*

~Adena C. E. Minott,
How to Be Beautiful and Keep Youthful (1923) from Part II,
Growing Beautiful Metaphysically

While I'm applying my creams and oil I say two Our Fathers and two Hail Marys. I tell God, "You've just got to help me take care of my face and neck!" I say it imploringly, not demandingly. My faith, I've been told, is childlike. This was not, I believe, intended as a compliment. But I cannot fault it. I do think of God as my father.

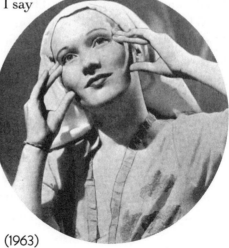

~Hildegarde,
Over 50—So What! (1963)

When a friendly young woman discovers that she is growing wrinkles, there is something wrong . . .

Heavy cream is applied at night with light, brisk, tapping of the finger ends will so tone the tissues of the face that light wrinkles evaporate. A round and round motion is likely to push the flesh upward toward the eyes, causing turkey tracks. While the cream remains on the skin, iron with ice. Say prayers and go to bed.

~Helen Follett Jameson,
The Beauty Box (1931)

Every time I was complimented, I said, "Thank you, Lord," and affirmed, "IT IS TRUE, I AM THAT."

When you meet a pretty person with a strong personality, don't feel like a worm in the dust of his or her presence. Throw your head back, straighten your shoulders, visualize yourself as you wish to be, and say silently, and feel, "I am just as beautiful and impressive as she. The same God that lives in her lives in me, and is no respecter of persons." That will pull you out and give you poise. We can't have low, evil thoughts on the inside and reflect virtue and beauty outside. The Bible says our thoughts and conversations are heard aloud in heaven. They are also heard and seen on our countenance. "As man thinketh in his heart, so is he." Remember, thoughts are like mosquitos. Watch your screens.

Put away from thee a wayward mouth and perverse lips. Weigh carefully the path of thy feet and let all thy way be ordered aright. —Prov. 20-27

Sincere desire is prayer. But God will not hear a wicked prayer, or one that will harm anyone else. Praying for beauty in order to lord it over someone else, or to make someone else envious is a wicked prayer. But praying to be more pleasing to people's eyes and to make one more useful is God's will. God loves beauty. Look at the beauty of nature God has made.

~Edith Carter,
From Duckling to Swan (1948)

A powder of magic property, handed down in the "Marquise de Fontenoy's" family from an ancestress who was a celebrated beauty at the court of Louis XIV, is prepared in this manner.

Poudre D'amour
    Scrape six juicy, raw carrots and half a pink beetroot, squeeze the juice out through a muslin bag, and put it aside. Take three ounces finely powdered

cornstarch, mix with the carrot and the beet juice, expose it to the sun, and stir occasionally until the fluid evaporates, leaving the tinted starch dry.

~Ella Adelia Fletcher,
The Woman Beautiful (1901)

A Powder to Prevent
Baldness
Powder your head with
powdered Parsley Seed, at night, once in
three or four months, and the hair will never
fall off.

~The Toilet of Flora
(originally published in 1779, reissued in 1939)

I shall never be more than twenty, as I firmly believe in that familiar phrase 'A woman is as old as she looks,' and that I look twenty and always shall, is my reason for writing this book.

~Edna Wallace Hopper,
My Secrets of Youth and Beauty (1925)

I am utterly convinced that this sunlight nutrition diet will help every human ill, excepting only the results of an

This Modern Fad

I found references to "the raw food faddists" that dated as far back as the mid-1800s. Ms. Rubinstein had a restaurant and health institute in New York City devoted to the raw diet at the time her book came out. It was all the rage. She is no less evangelical than today's raw foodists. I was, however, surprised to note just how much cream cheese Ms. Rubinstein's diet included.

accident or some organic malformation. That statement will startle you. I want it to startle you. Then you will pay heed and set your feet now on the path to beautiful young health. There are two things every woman prays for. One is a flawless skin. The other is a healthy slender body. But before she can have either, she must realize that vital cleanliness is the basis on which they are built. By vital cleanliness I mean that she must be utterly free of constipation. I mean that she can banish pills, oils, mineral salts, abdominal massage and other temporary remedies from her day. A normally functioning system will not need such artificial aids. When she has learned to follow this beautifying diet of raw fruits and vegetables, she will discover that a properly fed body functions normally.

~Helena Rubinstein,
Food for Beauty (1938)

Every woman, regardless of age, owes to herself, her public, and her Creator a well-proportioned, lithe and graceful figure.

~Mary Jane Moore, R.N.,
You Can Too! (1950)

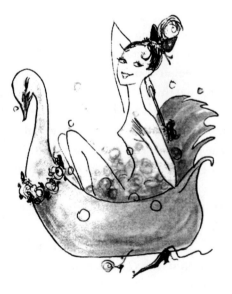

Even a crooked nose may be straightened by persistent manipulation during childhood, but this will not avail much in later life. If your nose be oily or shiny, bathe occasionally with weak borax water, or dust with rice powder, prepared chalk or magnesium. Do not cultivate a scornful attitude toward life in general. It finds its unbeautiful physical reflex in a habitual elevation of the nostrils in a most disagreeable manner.

~Florence Courtenay,
Physical Beauty (1922)

We have all heard of the woman who declared that, "The sense of being well dressed gives a feeling of inward tranquility which religion is powerless to bestow." Courage and clothes have so much to do with one another. A well-ordered dress helps to put one at leisure from one's self. The ease of it, the sense of fitness it induces, prepare the mind for the right attitude of courtesy to others.

~Francis Mary Steele and **Elizabeth Livingston Steele Adams,**
Beauty of Form and Grace of Vesture (1892)

In America there is a superstition about yellow garters being exceedingly lucky. I do not know how far the truth of this assertion goes, but I confess that primrose garters clasped with topaz mounted in burnished gold are a very attractive adjunct to the feminine toilette. In my humble opinion, the prettiest of all garters are the black, ruched with Chantilly lace, and fastened by a buckle made of tiny brilliants, for wear with black silk hose, and garters of a shade to match that of the stockings for the evening. A detail which should never be omitted is to sew a tiny sachet on the inside of each garter.

~The Marquise de Fontenoy,
Eve's Glossary (1897)

His Satanic Majesty ought not to have a monopoly of pretty clothes any more than he should of all the good times and good tunes.

~Belle Armstrong Whitney,
What to Wear (1916)

It is one of the sad and accepted facts of fashion life that clothes will look their best on you if your waistline is about 26". (Later we'll tell you how to make it look nearer this figure if it isn't.)

If you are on the plump side, you will be amazed to find what a Scheherezade world is opened to you when you lose weight.

~Bea Danville,
Dress Well on $1 a Day (1956)

You may readily understand why it is of value when ever sipping water to accompany the act with the thought: *With every sip of water I drink I shall think, this is to increase the action of the bowels* (place your hand over your bowels). *Tomorrow morning at* (select a convenient time and keep every engagement with yourself) *they will move freely, freely and naturally.*

~Alice M. Long,
My Lady Beautiful (1908)

Believe it or not, doctors are still saying that the first thing to do is to find a wart-charmer, because warts do behave in the most extraordinarily unpredictable way. The power of suggestion seems to work on them. Beating them with a holly leaf and murmuring incantations is as effective, often, as the various wart solvents.

~Kate Morland,
The Book of the Body (1971)

A beautiful mind irradiates and gives loveliness. You can cultivate it. Wipe out from your mind all thoughts and ideas not in keeping with true beauty, for on the face are often written the thoughts and ideas that run through you, and if they are ugly and undesirable you can be pretty sure you are not conveying to the world a happy, kind and lovely face.

~How to Attain and Retain Beauty (1935)

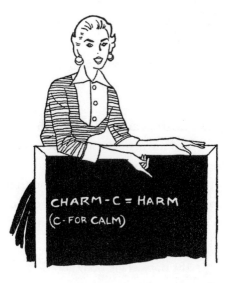

Because I Said So

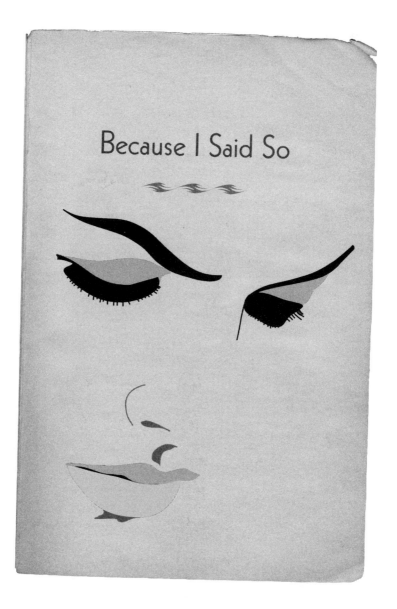

Why false eyelashes are indispensable, how measurement charts to the quarter inch guarantee failure, and, of course, what one must wear for hunting. Find out the importance of hammering yourself into classical proportion and why a permanent is a must for every woman. In short, arbitrary rules from domineering experts.

One has to make her own body as nearly as possible like the classic models, by exercise, by diet, by every healthful process, or, as a last resort, to simulate corresponding proportions by every harmless device of art in clothing.

~Francis Mary Steele and **Elizabeth Livingston Steele Adams,**
Beauty of Form and Grace of Vesture (1892)

You must learn to make up your eyes with shadow and painted-on liner, and to wear false eyelashes as inevitably as ordinary girls wear panties.

~Jean Rook,
Dressing for Success (1968)

THE OVERWEIGHT WOMAN SHOULD NEVER WEAR SLACKS.

The unfortunate part of wearing slacks is that we ourselves are never aware of just what we look like in them. Somehow the mirror does not show us the back view in its real appearance and perspective; if the overweight woman could ever see the rear of her self in slacks, she would never put them on again. If she feels she must wear them to work in her garden or to work outside her house or inside at menial jobs to protect her, then let her take them off the moment she is through with her task.

Never for a moment should she imagine that she looks cute in them or that they are acceptable apparel, because they are not. From the standpoint of glamour, they are poison.

~Margery Wilson,
You're As Young As You Act (1951)

A Deportment which would become a short and thick-set woman would never do for one of a tall and slender figure, with a long neck and contracted waist. The woman of larger proportions may safely affect the majestic gait and air; but how absurd it would be for a tall and slender figure to stiffen her joints, throw back her head, and march off with a military air? The character of these light forms corresponds with their resemblances in the vegetable world. The poplar, the willow, and the graceful lily, bend their gentle heads at each passing breeze, and their flexible and tender arms toss in the wind with motions of grace and beauty. Such is the woman of delicate proportions. She must enter a room either with the buoyant step of a young nymph, if youth is her passport to sportiveness; or, if she is advanced nearer the meridian of life, she may glide in with that ease of manner which gives play to all the graceful motions of her undulating form. For her to crane up her neck would change its swanlike bend into the scraggy throat of an ostrich.

~Madame Lola Montez,
The Arts and Secrets of Beauty (1853)

TEN BEAUTY COMMANDMENTS

1. Thou shalt exercise faithfully and wisely at least once a day.
2. Thou shalt be ever fastidious and dainty in thy person.
3. Thou shalt be at all times groomed and prepared for public inspection.
4. Thou shalt strive for perfection of spirit and character, as well as surface beauty.
5. Thou shalt keep an open mind and a weather eye for any and all new beauty secrets.
6. Thou shalt plan a day which provides time for personal care, abundant rest and proper meals.

7. Thou shalt make the most of thy attractive features and seek to improve defective ones.

8. Thou shalt seek professional guidance in selecting full foundation garments.

9. Thou shalt choose thy costumes to become thyself, and not according to style trends.

10. Thou shalt keep thy goal of perfection ever in sight. And work toward it constantly.

~Joe Bonomo,
Figure Ritual no. 34 pamphlet (1965)

Your Correct Proportions

HEIGHT Ft. In.	WEIGHT Lbs.	BUST In.	WAIST In.	HIPS In.	NECK In.	ARM In.	THIGH In.	CALF In.
4-11	112- 1/2	30- 7/10	23- 3/5	32- 1/5	12- 1/5	9- 4/5	17- 3/4	12- 1/5
5	113- 1/2	31- 1/8	24	32- 3/5	12- 2/5	10	18	12- 2/5
5- 3/5	114- 1/2	31- 1/2	24- 2/5	33	12- 1/2	10- 1/10	18- 1/5	12- 1/2
5- 1-2/5	116- 3/4	31- 4/5	24- 4/5	33- 2/5	12- 3/5	10- 1/4	18- 1/2	12- 3/5
5- 2	119	32- 1/5	25- 1/5	33- 4/5	12- 4/5	10- 2/5	18- 3/4	12- 4/5
5- 3	123- 1/2	32- 3/5	25- 3/5	34- 1/4	13	10- 1/2	19	13
5- 3-4/5	125- 3/4	33	26	34- 3/5	13- 1/8	10- 3/5	19- 1/4	13- 1/7
5- 4-1/2	128	33- 2/5	26- 2/5	35	13- 1/3	10- 3/4	19- 1/2	13- 1/3
5- 5-1/3	131	33- 4/5	26- 4/5	35- 2/5	13- 2/5	10- 9/10	19- 4/5	13- 2/5
5- 6	133- 2/5	34- 1/4	27- 1/5	35- 4/5	13	11	20	13- 3/5
5- 7	137- 4/5	34- 3/5	27- 3/5	36- 1/5	13- 3/4	11- 1/10	20- 3/10	13- 3/4
5- 7-3/4	139	35	28	36- 3/5	13- 9/10	11- 1/4	20- 3/5	13- 9/10
5- 8-1/2	141	35- 2/5	28- 2/5	37	14	11- 2/5	20- 4/5	14
5- 9	145- 1/2	35- 4/5	28- 3/4	37- 2/5	14- 1/4	11- 1/2	21- 1/10	14- 1/4
5- 10	148- 4/5	36- 1/5	29- 1/8	37- 4/5	14- 2/5	11- 3/5	21- 2/5	14- 2/5
5- 11	151	36- 3/5	29- 1/2	38- 1/5	14- 3/5	11- 4/5	21- 3/5	14- 3/5

I bobbed my hair and I believe in it. I think it is the most universally becoming style of coiffure ever evolved. It is convenient and it is youthful. But there are bobs and bobs. I am not at all in favor of the bob which includes a shaved neck. I call this the "convict bob" and I think it disfiguring to any woman, young or old.

~Edna Hopper Wallace,
My Secrets of Youth and Beauty (1925)

Most women require permanents or at least part permanents, and there is no other beauty service which does more to bring out a woman's beauty and lift her morale than a good permanent if properly given.

~Hazel Theresa Gifford,
Fundamentals of Beauty (1944)

Mere plumpness is not beauty. True facial beauty is enhanced by lines of *artistic physical expression.* . . .

As a rule, French women are not beautiful, but the mobility of their lips in speech is most fascinating. Others may acquire this mobility and facility by the practice of labial exercises.

~Elizabeth Hubbard,
Beauty, How Acquired and Retained (1910)

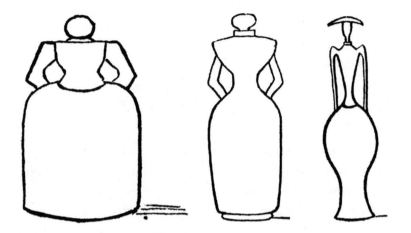

The rhythm of two lines diverging and converging is
most agreeable. We are conscious of this pleasure
when we follow the outlines of a vase, a newel post,
or a turret. The conventional, tailor-made figure of
today has undoubtedly these charms. Similar curves
in a stout woman may give the satisfaction we take in
the robust bulge of an odd jug, or the squat of a

quaintly shaped bottle. All this may be pleasing or otherwise in baked clay, but is out of place in a living woman.

~Francis Mary Steele and Elizabeth Livingston Steele Adams,
Beauty of Form and Grace of Vesture (1892)

The outward and visible bodily condition which precedes maternity is the last thing of which a woman should feel ashamed. It is indeed the sign of a glorious responsibility and should be revered as such. At the same time, it cannot be denied that an unavoidable distortion of the body is one of the results of the pregnancy, especially as it approaches in term. But the mother who has been thus blessed, need not, necessarily, "point with pride" to her condition. True pride is modest and does not try to make itself conspicuous.

~Florence Courtenay,
Physical Beauty (1922)

Is it in good taste to wear slacks around the streets of New York? This is a moot question, which arouses everyone to discussion. That makes it a good problem. Many women look messy in slacks. Their figures are not neat, and don't look neat in anything. Slacks conceal nothing. For such women, it is bad taste to wear slacks anywhere being neat takes first place. . . . [M]any women look very neat in slacks. . . . Some of them habitually wear slacks in New York when they walk their dogs in the park. During skiing season, hundreds of women pour through Grand Central Terminal, headed for the ski country in ski pants. All this seems to be in perfectly good taste.

~Elizabeth Hawes,
Good Grooming (1942)

Regardless of prevailing fashions, good taste demands that skirts for street wear never be worn shorter than one inch below the bend of the knee in back. Anything shorter than this only succeeds in removing all grace and impressiveness from a figure in motion.

~Dorothy Preble,
from Ern and Bud Westmore's Beauty, Glamour and Personality
(1947)

For forest shooting, where it is a question of going through thickets and brambles, the skirt should be replaced by breeches. These should be narrower and more close-fitting than riding breeches, and should be worn with small canvas and leather boots, "waders" made of unbleached waterproof linen, green or grey, and a short cloth coat matching in colour a small felt hat of neutral shade.

The whole should be of the utmost restraint. By a kind of inverted snobbery, it is accepted that the more shabby these garments look, the more elegant they are. The outfit should include a short poplin raincoat.

The male uniform is exactly the same — men and women are indistinguishable when out shooting — except that, of course, trousers or breeches take the place of skirts.

~Jacqueline Du Pasquier,
A Guide to Elegance (1956)

If You Live In Town. If you are a career girl living in the city, you must gradually gather together in your glove drawer the following: one pair of everyday gloves in a long wearing leather; one pair of white "shorties" in cotton or nylon fabric; one pair of elbow-length black or dark-colored suede to match your dark clothes, one pair of woolen, pigskin, or string gloves for sports and informal wear.

~Bea Danville,
Dress Well on $1 a Day (1956)

I DO NOT THINK THE OLDER WOMAN
SHOULD SLIDE INTO WHAT WE CALL THE
STOLID, MATRONLY CLOTHES UNTIL SHE IS
FINISHED WITH DANCING.

I think that's a good time to measure the change by.

~Margery Wilson,
You're As Young As You Act (1951)

Meat, Grease, and Booze

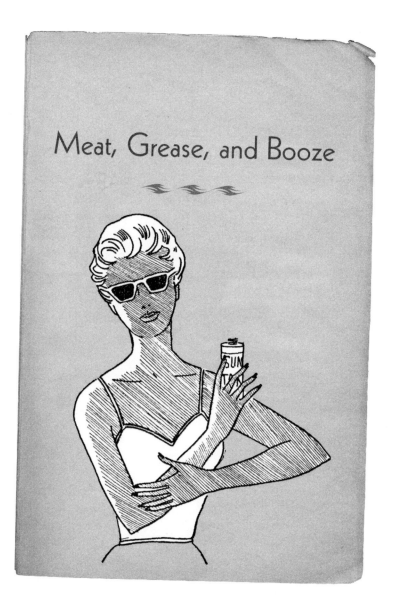

~

Remarkably, meat-based beauty tips are no joke. In this chapter:
what not to bathe in, more mentions of mutton than is prudent,
and why taking to your bed with a stiff drink is probably the cure for
whatever ails you. Become schooled in condiments for beauty.
Learn the history of Vaseline, and meet its most devoted enthusiasts.
Expect revulsion, incredulity, and horror-movie screams.

~

There are all kinds of masks, ranging from the simplest of clay packs to the meat mask. . . . Fresh beef is cut into very thin slices, according to a pattern you should make at home. Cut pieces out of paper—a strip to cover the forehead, another for cheeks, chin and a thin narrow strip for the nose. Give your pattern to the butcher who will cut the meat accordingly. Leave openings around the eyes and lips. Pack the meat over your skin and secure it with a strip of muslin which has also been cut according to pattern. Leave it on for one or two hours or overnight if possible.

~Helena Rubinstein,
The Art of Feminine Beauty (1930)

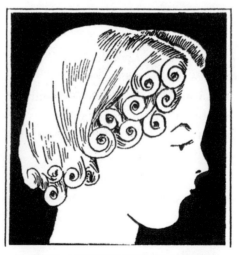

HOW TO ARRANGE THE PIN CURLS.

For slightly faded ladies, I am a great believer in a glass of red wine at least once a day with lunch or dinner, and every night and morning a good massage with pure turtle oil.

~Jane Gordon,
Home Beauty Treatments (1943)

If you like liquor, have it straight. Mixed drinks add calories and fluid. A straight whiskey will get you where you want to be as quickly as a Manhattan, and you'll be thinner when you get there.

~Polly Bergen,
Polly's Principles (1974)

Face Butter Moisturizing Cream
    1 container any brand margarine
    That's all. Margarine is already a solidified mixture of oils (note soy oil on package) which works wonderfully as a moisturizer for women who don't care to make their own.

~Alexandra York,
Back to Basics Natural Beauty Handbook (1977)

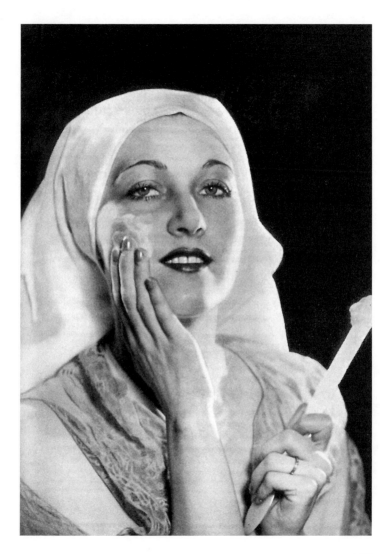

Have ready some soft pomatum of beef marrow, boiled with a little almond or olive oil, flavored with a mild perfume. Rub a small quantity of this on the skin of the head after it has been washed as above. This may be efficient, but in this age, women prefer the cleanlier method of stimulating the hair without pomade.

~Mrs. Susan C. D. Power,
The Ugly-Girl Papers (1874)

The best remedy for the cure of dandruff is the unguent known under the name of the "Dupuytren Recipe":

Take of	
Beef marrow	11 ounces
Acetate of lead,	60 grains.
Black balsam of Peru,	300 "
Rectified alcohol,	2 fluid ounces.
Cantharide powder,	25 grains.
Essence of clover,	10 drops
Essence of Cinnamon,	10 drops

~The Marquise de Fontenoy,
Eve's Glossary (1897)

One of the finest hair tonics, if not the best one known, is this:

> 1 pt. High Wine
> 1 pt. Water
> 1 oz. Bear's Oil

By applying it to the scalp, it not only stops the hair falling out, almost at the first application, but it will restore gray hair to its natural color, and cause the hair to thicken.

High Wine is alcohol before it is distilled. Do not allow a druggist to give you poor whiskey for high wine, as a great many will do. High Wine can only be found at a distillery, and cannot be bought, as it is not stamped. Sometimes a distiller, out of the kindness of his heart, will give it to you.

~Amy Ayer,
Facts for Ladies (1908)

A little refined beef marrow rubbed gently into the hair roots is a good natural tonic (though an old-fashioned one) and together with plenty of fresh air and sunshine, does more for the hair than all the compounded tonics and "restorers" marketed.

~Florence Courtenay,
Physical Beauty (1922)

Vaseline Conditioner: For really dry or damaged hair, this old home remedy can't be beat. It takes several shampooings to wash out, though, so don't make the mistake of once-over-lightly and expecting your hair to look lovely. You'll have to scrub more than usual after this treatment. Soften a couple of tablespoons of Vaseline over a double boiler and then combine with a teaspoon of Ivory Flakes. Mix together in a blender or with an electric beater until frothy and white. Use this like one of those deep conditioners that you put on your hair and leave for at least twenty minutes. For additional benefits, wrap a hot towel around your hair. As I said, you'll have to shampoo several times to get the Vaseline out, but the results will be worth the effort.

~Gloria Richards,
A New You (1980)

Vaseline is a byproduct of the petroleum drilling process. It was discovered in Pennsylvania in 1859, by Brooklynite Robert Cheesebrough. While working on a rig, he became fascinated by the greasy substance that clogged the pumps. Workers had noticed it seemed to help skin heal quicker. Soon, Robert was distributing the stuff all over New York, and thus began his empire.

Many Parisian ladies, in the secrecy of their chambers, on retiring at night, or some part of the day, bind their faces with thin slices of raw beef or veal. For several years a popular lady of the "American colony" in Paris, has used this remedy to feed the tissues of the face, with remarkable results. At thirty-eight she has the complexion and skin of a girl of eighteen. It may not be pleasant to contemplate, but it prevents and removes wrinkles as nothing else will. Other ladies noted for their fine complexions, sleep in masks made of rubber or silk.

~Amy Ayer,
Facts for Ladies (1908)

Those who wish to gain flesh and those who need fatty matter but whose stomachs do not take kindly to its digestion derive great advantage from massaging with oil after the Turkish bath. For this purpose many oils are used . . . Olive, cocoa-nut, cotton-seed, almond, and even cod-liver oils have their advocates."

~Elle Adelia Fletcher,
The Woman Beautiful (1901)

Both Spanish and French women — those at least who are very particular to make the most of these charms — are in the habit of sleeping in gloves which are lined or plastered over with a kind of pomade to improve the delicacy and complexion of their hands. This paste is generally made of the following ingredients.

Take a half pound of soft soap, a gill of salad oil, an ounce of mutton tallow, and boil then until they are thoroughly mixed. After the boiling has ceased, but before it is cold, add one gill of spirits of wine, and a grain of musk.

If any lady wishes to try this she can buy a pair of gloves three or four sizes larger than the hand, rip them open and spread on this layer of the paste, and then sew the gloves up again. There is no doubt that by wearing them every night they will give smoothness and a fine complexion to the hands. Those who have the means, can send to Paris and purchase them ready made. But I am not aware that they have been imported to this country. It will not surprise me, however, to learn that they have been, for fashionable ladies are remarkably quick at finding out the tricks which the belles elsewhere resort to for the purpose of beautifying themselves.

~Madame Lola Montez,
The Arts and Secrets of Beauty (1853)

In the eighteenth century, the ladies of the nobility wanted milk baths . . . of almond paste, of flesh water (in which veal had been boiled). . . . These were undeniably good for the skin; but cleanliness does not require all these accessories. . . . A strong concoction of spinach also makes an excellent bath.

~**Harriet Hubbard Ayer,**
My Lady's Dressing Room (1892)

Vaseline has the valuable quality of never growing rancid; it acts like a charm against slight eruptions, or rash from disturbed circulation, and it is an unequalled lubricator of the knees and other joints while exercising.

~**Ella Adelia Fletcher,**
The Woman Beautiful (1901)

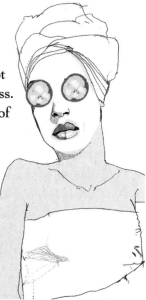

Whiskey in the Tub: A friend of mine swears by this one, and even though it's not on the diet, I've included it for completeness. Try it after you get thin. Just take a jigger of whiskey, a jigger of lemon juice in which you've dissolved a suitable amount of sugar, mix them together in a glass, and take the whole concoction into the tub where you—yes, drink it. Slowly. While you steep. Not for every day, even when you're not dieting, but relaxing, for sure.

~**Gloria Richards,**
A New You (1980)

Portuguese woman are said to get satisfactory results from the following simple treatment:

Boil two whole small oranges in a pint of olive oil for three to four hours—the boiling must to be done in a water jacket, that is, the oil and oranges are put in a pan set inside of another pan that contains the water. At night, a piece of the boiled orange is gently rubbed over the bust. A few weeks' treatment, it is said, makes the bust much firmer and harder.

~William A. Woodbury,
Beauty Culture (1910)

For a softer skin, rub rich sour cream into your body before you take a shower, then let the water rinse it away.

~Barbara Walden,
Easy Glamour (1981)

Exercise No. 9

Stand with feet well apart, whole body relaxed, arms hanging loosely. Now shake the body, only gently, using the least possible muscular exertion, until conscious of a feeling of general muscle relaxation and restfulness. This exercise may be varied by walking about, allowing the whole body to sway and sag, as if deeply intoxicated.

~Sarah C. Turner,
The Attainment of Womanly Beauty (1900)

Of cold creams, there are numerous good sorts—
Vaseline cold cream, olive oil, rose ointment, lemon
cream—these all come under the same head. Do not
try to make your own skin food; buy a standard
preparation.

~**Ella Adelia Fletcher,**
The Woman Beautiful (1901)

The following pomade will help if rubbed over the fatty
parts twice a day:

Iodide of Potassium	50 gr.
Vaseline	2 oz
Lanolin	2 oz
Tincture of Benzoin	25 drops

Exercise, however, is the best means of bust reduction.

~**William A. Woodbury,**
Beauty Culture (1910)

Reducing Dressing (1 pint)
1 ½ cup chemically pure mineral oil
⅛ strained lemon juice
1 teaspoon vegetable salt
2 saccharine tablets

½ egg yolk
1 small sliver fresh garlic if desired.

~Helena Rubinstein,
Food for Beauty (1938)

Sometimes little black specks appear about the base of
the nose, or on the forehead, or in the hollow of the chin,
which are called "fleshworms," and are occasioned by
coagulated lymph that obstructs the pores of the skin.
They may be pressed out by pressing the skin, and
ignorant people suppose them to be little worms. They
are permanently removed by washing with warm water,
and severe friction with a towel, and then applying a
little of the following preparation:

Liquor of potassa . . .	1 oz.
Cologne	1 oz.
White brandy	1 oz.

~Madame Lola Montez,
The Arts and Secrets of Beauty (1853)

The eyelashes may be improved by delicately cutting off
their forked and gossamer points, and anointing with a
salve of two drachms of ointment of nitric oxide of

mercury and one drachm of lard. Mix the lard and ointment well, and anoint the edges of the eyelids night and morning, washing after each time with warm milk and water. This, it is said, will restore the lashes when lost by disease.

~Mrs. Susan C. D. Power,
The Ugly-Girl Papers (1874)

I am often asked why actors and actresses preserve their clearness of complexion better than most people. The reason is to be found in the free use of oil and fatty substances employed in making up. I may perhaps interest some of my readers to know how this is done.

[A] good base for make-up is rendered lard, made by pouring boiling water on lard in a basin. The water goes to the bottom and the lard remains on the top, mingled with as much water as it can hold. It is then skimmed off, put in a cloth and any excess water squeezed out. It is usually scented with oil verbena, though attar of roses is pleasanter, but more expensive.

~Cora Brown Potter,
The Secrets of Beauty and Mysteries of Health (1908)

A flesh-making cream, which may be used when the face is thin, is made from two and a half ounces of lanoline, a quarter of an ounce of spermaceti, two and a half ounces

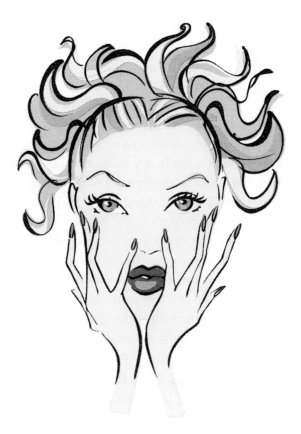

of freshly dried mutton tallow, two ounces each of cocoanut oil and oil of sweet almonds, half a dram of tincture of benzoin, and ten drops of neroli.

~Margaret Mixter,
Health and Beauty Hints (1910)

Chapped Lips. — A simple, easily made remedy is a combination of mutton or lamb tallow and camphor. Melt a piece of gum camphor about the size of a walnut with two ounces of the tallow. Keep in a porcelain or glass jar.

~William A. Woodbury,
Beauty Culture (1910)

The best massage oil for the face is good old Vaseline. (I strongly suspect that someday it will be proven that Vaseline contains some secret ingredient that makes it superior to some of the most expensive creams, but it hasn't happened yet.) To make the Vaseline easier for the skin to absorb — so you won't look like you're greased up to swim the English Channel when you're done — heat a few tablespoons in the top of a double boiler until it melts. If you want to smell good, add a few drops of your favorite perfume. No scent clashes with Vaseline.

~Gloria Richards,
A New You (1980)

One of the most important points in making up is to carefully cleanse the skin before and after this operation with very pure white vaseline, which in some measure prevents painting from becoming too irritating.

~The Marquise de Fontenoy,
Eve's Glossary (1897)

The only safe and astringent "oily" unguent for the skin is mutton suet refined and slightly perfumed. It should be applied from neck to heels with the hand and gently rubbed in so as not to shine or become sticky. It then leaves a soft, satiny surface. This treatment prevents layers of fat from forming under the skin, and stout people will be surprised to see how rapidly it will reduce their bulk if continued nightly.

~The Marquise de Fontenoy,
Eve's Glossary (1897)

Mix two parts lemon juice to one part Jamaica rum, and pat on freckles. (I suppose you can drink what's left over, and then you won't *care* whether you have freckles or not!)

~Deborah Rutledge,
Natural Beauty Secrets (1969)

Arts and Crafts

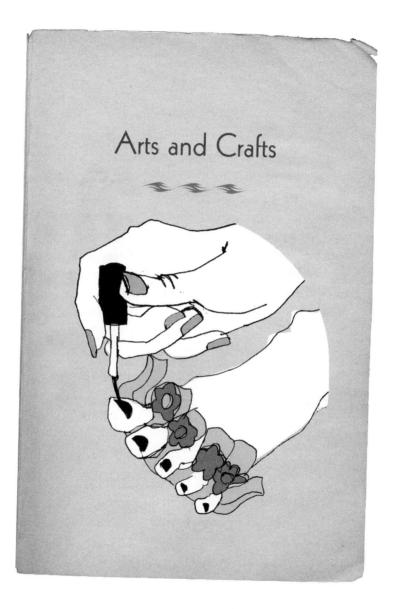

Smoke, mirrors, and projects for when you have way too much free time. Here are the domestic dark arts, including alternate uses for rolling pins and mops, and truly painterly makeup. These authors were industrious and determined. They took tips from both art school and the kitchen, and were willing to put in the elbow grease to make it all work. Think of this chapter as a beauty manual by Martha Stewart.

Use liquid powder on the hands if they are red, or green powder may be used on them to complete an evening toilet. This gives red hands an elegant and ethereal appearance.

~Sonya Joslen,
The Way to Beauty (1937)

Bright crimson silk dipped in spirits of wine and rubbed upon the cheeks, chin, and ears is said to be a safe and harmless rouge that defies detection. It requires all the skill of a portrait painter—a deft touch with the fingers and a skillful eye—to make up so that you impose upon even the most indifferent eye. And any makeup which is not discreetly and artistically managed is vulgar in the extreme.

~Ella Adelia Fletcher,
The Woman Beautiful (1901)

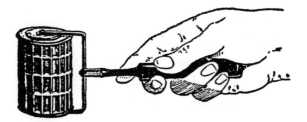

Any stubborn lump of flesh can be squeezed off. . . . [I]t works perfectly well on all parts of the body, hips, thighs, waist, anywhere in fact except the breasts. Never squeeze or massage the breasts.

First, cover your hands with massaging cream. Take up handfuls of flesh, squeeze hard, then let it slip through your fingers like mashed potatoes. You can squeeze off fat cells in this manner. . . . After squeezing, put a Turkish towel over the part you're reducing and slap good and hard.

~Sylvia of Hollywood,
No More Alibis (1934)

Now that a great many households are coming to depend on the corner grocery for cookies and pastries, the old-fashioned rolling pin is facing a decline. True, it still figures as a symbol of wifely authority in our comic strips, but its original work, that of smoothing flat soft masses of dough, is now little in demand in many homes.

A new use, however, has been found for the rolling pin. This humble implement of the domestic arts has been adapted to the noble work of beautifying milady's figure, by massaging away the superfluous fat on limbs, neck, back and abdomen. It should not be used on breasts for fear of bruising them.

~Lois Leeds,
Beauty and Health (1927)

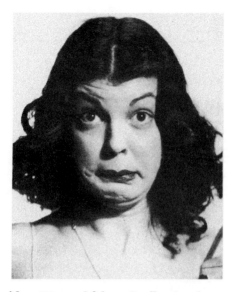

No. 73 — (Above) To develop muscles of the jaw, neck and chest & prevent wrinkles in forehead and around eyes. Draw down corners of mouth, at the same time stretching eyes open as wide as possible. Then clench jaws together.

Wrinkles? Oil 'em and freeze 'em. At night apply a heavy emollient, slap the face briskly, hammer it with finger tips. Sponge on an astringent, skate over the celestial countenance with a piece of ice. In the morning use more ice.

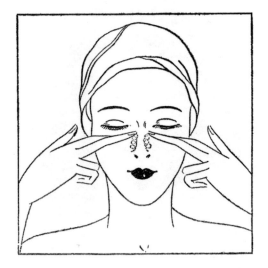

Heavy cream applied at night with light, brisk, tapping of the finger ends will so tone the tissues of the face that light wrinkles evaporate. A round and round motion is likely to push the flesh upward toward the eyes, causing turkey tracks. While the cream remains on the skin, iron with ice. Say prayers and go to bed. In the morning use ice again. . . .

~Helen Follett Jameson,
The Beauty Box (1931)

Many of the ordinary household duties, such as wielding the humdrum floor mop, may be transformed into exercises for beautifying the hips and waist. This exercise can be performed by drawing the figure into an erect position as the mop is brought towards the body.

~Sonya Joslen,
The Way to Beauty (1937)

Do you wear your hair in an upsweep? Rouge your earlobes, by all means. Illness or too much dieting can sometimes make earlobes pale and waxy looking, which suggests ill health. A touch of pink and you're not only glowing but your earrings, should you wear them, will be more dramatic.

~Rita Gam,
The Beautiful Woman (1967)

Leg Make-up: When you use leg make-up, apply a thin coat of mineral oil first and let it dry. Then spread papers on the floor so you won't splatter make-up. Allow yourself at least ten minutes to do the job right.

1. Start make-up at the instep and smooth upward to a point above the knee. Be sure to end it in an even line. Tie a ribbon

around your thigh where the "stocking" ends and remove it when make-up dries.

2. Pat make-up with the palms of your hands, then buff with cotton. Inspect the backs of the legs, too, to be sure they're even.

3. Never try to patch up yesterday's make-up job. Besides, leg make-up is drying to the skin and should be thoroughly washed off every night.

4. Be careful if you cross your legs on hot summer days not to smudge your make-up.

~Babs Lee,
ABC's of Beauty (1950)

Detachable sleeves are a good ruse for converting an afternoon frock into a dinner dress. The sleeves, which are kept in place by elastic run through the top and slipped over the shoulder, are pulled off as easily as a glove.

Another good dress transformation is a garden party frock that is also an evening gown . . . The over-dress is of net of chiffon or organdie, and when this is removed a perfectly cut slip of heavy silk faille is revealed.

~How to Attain and Retain Beauty (1935)

Dry Shampoos
CORN MEAL AND SALT

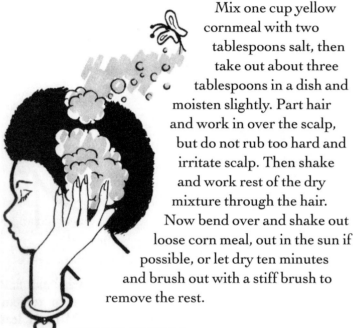

Mix one cup yellow cornmeal with two tablespoons salt, then take out about three tablespoons in a dish and moisten slightly. Part hair and work in over the scalp, but do not rub too hard and irritate scalp. Then shake and work rest of the dry mixture through the hair. Now bend over and shake out loose corn meal, out in the sun if possible, or let dry ten minutes and brush out with a stiff brush to remove the rest.

WHITE OF EGG

Beat white of two eggs stiff. Part hair and put both on scalp and hair. A small nail brush is good to use to get down to strands of hair. Be sure it is completely dry before starting to brush out.

~Hazel Theresa Gifford,
Fundamentals of Beauty (1944)

Most necks need regular bleaching treatments to make the skin smooth and white enough to be presentable in an evening gown. To make them so, they must be scrubbed thoroughly each night with pure soap and warm water. A fairly stiff bath brush should be used for this purpose. This method of cleansing has the double advantage of stimulating the circulation and removing scarfskin and grime.

Notice how a pink flush replaces the sallowness of the neck after massage or scrubbing. Unless special pains are taken to stimulate the flow of blood here the skin tends to become flabby and yellow.

After the lathering and scrubbing, the parts should be thoroughly rinsed in clear, warm water, then in cold and finally dried very carefully. In place of the cold rinse, buttermilk may be used to lighten the skin color. Leave this bleach on for half an hour before rinsing it all off.

~**Lois Leeds,**
Beauty and Health (1927)

If your lips are too thin, line just outside the natural lip line. If they are too thick, line just inside the natural lip line. Then draw an inverted V in the center of your upper lip and a regular V on the bottom lip. Draw several vertical lines around both top and bottom lips. Finally, fill in with your matching lipstick. The lines will not show at all. Blot up, reapply, and blot lightly. Your lipstick will stay stuck for hours.

~Linda Stasi,
Looking Good is the Best Revenge (1984)

Blending is not simply a case of fading out a flat, constant color. Think of the way light strikes a curved surface, such as a cup or saucer. When a surface curves outward, you see a gradation of dark to light to dark. On the concave surface, it is just the reverse: light to dark to light. If you approach your face composition in terms of rounded areas and angles, following the "cup and saucer" school of blending, you will create a far more natural effect. You should never create a dark shadow without highlighting at least one side of it. And never use highlighting without adding a corresponding shadow to soften it.

~Diana Lewis Jewell,
Making Up by Rex (1986)

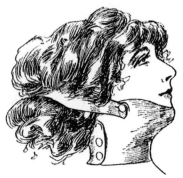

Chin-Chin Strap
(a secret weapon in the war against sags)
  This device can help enormously when it is supplemented by exercise. It

will whittle away soft underchin fat deposits and bring out your youthful, firm chin line. It is especially helpful for loose skin and hanging jowls.

Here is how to make a chin strap:

1. Fold a soft cotton handkerchief in half so a triangle is formed.
2. Spray face, neck, and underchin with mineral-water spray.
3. Attach a strong rubber band to the two ends at the base of the triangle and adjust the device so that the cloth handkerchief is under your chin and is held taut by the rubber band circling to the top of your head.
4. Adjust for a comfortable but tight pulling motion.
5. Pull the handkerchief down slightly and place a small piece of plastic wrap between the handkerchief and your skin. (The kind of plastic used in bags is fine.)
6. Replace the handkerchief against your underchin.
7. Wear the device as often as possible. You can even sleep in it if you find it comfortable enough.

Note: I like chin straps made of gum rubber; however, you can fashion any number of workable devices from elastic, rubber, plastic, or stretch fabric. The important thing is that the device support your underchin with slight pressure in order to discourage fat deposits.

~M.R. Saffon,
Youthlift (1981)

For older women who do not feel the need of a conventional facelift but who now and then feel the urge to look much younger for special occasions, I recommend what is known as the instant facelift, a Rube Goldberg contraption of gauze, glue, and elastic bands that you can buy or do yourself. If you live in or near a big city, just go to a place that sells theatrical makeup and ask for an instant facelift.

You make it in two sections: first the eye lift, then the chin lift. For the eyes, cut two small (about one-inch) pie-shaped wedges of gauze. Sew a strip of very narrow elastic tape to the narrow edge of each wedge. Glue one wedge of gauze directly in front of one ear, right under the hairline, with the narrower part of the wedge pointing upward toward the top of your head. When the two wedges with their elastic bands are well anchored, pull the bands up high and tight and tie them together at the back of your head, cutting off the excess.

Your biggest problem may be finding the kind of glue that will stick to your face. I had a special glue made for me when I was doing instant facelifts for Hedda Hopper and Marion Davies and many other Hollywood stars. If you have trouble finding a glue that works, try making your wedges with Band-Aids or other strong tape recommended by your druggist or theatrical supply house.

For the chin lift the gauze or tape should be attached just below and behind the ear lobe. Again, pull the elastic up tight and tie at the back of the head. You can sew hooks and eyes on the ends of the elastic if you know the exact length you need.

It's really simple once you get the knack of it—and find the proper glue or tape that won't come unstuck.

I do not recommend wearing instant facelifts all the time, but for short periods of time they can be marvelous picker-uppers for older women.

~George Masters,
The Masters Way to Beauty (1977)

The first things to consider are the lips. From very ancient times lemon has been the favorite means of promoting their redness; a slice of lemon or lime daily rubbed on the lips just to cause tingling leaves them pleasantly red, provided that they are not cracked.

~Cora Brown Potter,
The Secrets of Beauty and Mysteries of Health (1908)

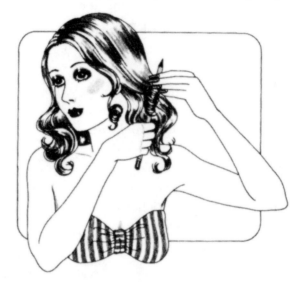

EYE MAKE-UP FOR STREET WEAR
To give the eyes a wonderful and attractive appearance, take an ordinary soft-lead pencil, darken the lower lid at the eyelash line, then apply mascara on the tips of the lashes.

~J. Ellsworth Hope,
The Art of Feminine Charm (1933)

One ounce of prepared horseradish you can buy at your grocers' and one pint of buttermilk. Simmer together over low heat for about an hour, stirring so it won't burn. Strain and then apply with cotton wool, but don't get it in your eyes. It's supposed to sting like anything.

~**Deborah Rutledge,**
Natural Beauty Secrets (1969)

Eau de cologne is a useful toilet accessory. Takes off the buttered look from too-oily hair. Rub into the scalp and dry the hair strand by strand with an old absorbent towel. Used on the complexion after the scrubbing and before the creaming it acts as an astringent and cleanser. Friction into the skin when gooseflesh is present.

~**Helen Follett,**
The Beauty Box (1931)

A cupful of curdled milk, poured into the hair and washed out, cleans it thoroughly and gives it the silken air of dark, falling water.

~**The Book of Indian Beauty** (1981)

A last-thing-at-night beauty pack that can be recommended is the lemon pack, which you can use about three times a week. Take a few slices of a fresh, juicy lemon, and from them extract the juice. Then add some olive oil in the proportion of a teaspoonful to each tablespoon of the juice, and put in enough oatmeal to make a paste which you should apply to the face. Leave it on all night, and in the morning remove with warm water and oatmeal. This is excellent for a dry skin.

~From **How to Attain and Retain Beauty**
(1935) from the Home Library of Great Britain

An important food staple in China and Japan is called tofu, or bean curd. This low-calorie, protein- and vitamin-packed, white cheese-like food (available in health-food and Asian food shops) makes a nourishing facial masque. Put half a block of bean curd in your blender with a quarter cup of milk and blend until smooth. Apply thickly to your face and leave for twenty minutes. Presto! The smooth, closely pored skin our Asian sisters are famous for is yours!

~**Barbara Walden,**
Easy Glamour (1981)

Take a piece of white cardboard, about 5" x 8". Look in the mirror and hold it up so that it covers one side of your face vertically, so that one eye shows, one nostril and one-half your lips. Look at that image.
Now place the cardboard on the other side of your face—and look again. Quite different, isn't it?

Does one side of your mouth look prettier, fuller, livelier, happier? Make that side up first, then make up the other side to match it! It's easy.

~Stan Place,
Stan Place's Guide to Makeup (1981)

When your ambition is satisfied, and hair of a "golden hue" has lost its charm, then it is time a full realization of "he who dances must pay the fiddler" comes in. If the hair has not commenced to fall out, and cutting close to the head is a positive necessity, it is better to do so at once, otherwise the colors of Joseph's coat would be few in comparison with the colors the hairs of the head will take on in its struggles to get back to nature's color.

~Amy Ayer,
Facts for Ladies (1908)

Mad Science

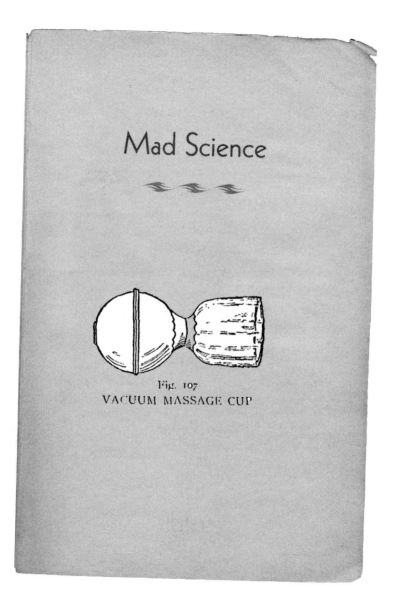

Fig. 107
VACUUM MASSAGE CUP

✦

Crackpot sugar theories, facial reconfiguring machines, and beauty in the Atomic Age. Call it **Better Looking Through Chemistry**. These tips are for all the department store beauty counter girls who have to wear lab coats. Read about plans to patent a personal sprinkler system for fresher complexions. And finally: introducing the inflatable bra.

✦

For scalp treatments, the up-to-date shop may have an assortment of electrical massage devices. The high frequency current is often used, applied to the scalp in a glass electrode, sometimes in the shape of a comb, inside which it sparkles and crackles with a purplish light, causing it to be termed violet ray.

~Edith Porter Lapish and **Flora G.Orr,**
Be Beautiful (1932)

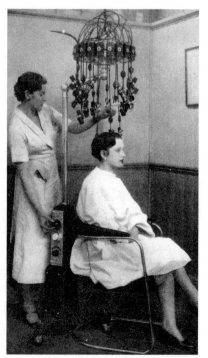

Think of the potent chemistry which awaits outside our windows untried! Among the list of "eyebrow pencils," "nail polishes," and lip salves, a foreign paper brings to notice one invention which might be of use—a nose-machine, which, we are told, so directs the soft cartilage that an ill-formed nose is quickly shaped to perfection. No surgeon will deny this is possible to a great degree. That it would be a boon nobody can doubt, seeing how many unfortunates walk the world whose noses have every appearance of having been sat upon, or made acquainted with the nether millstone.

~**Mrs. Susan C. D. Power,**
The Ugly-Girl Papers (1874)

The best effects of a shampoo can never be gained on cloudy, damp, or rainy days. The sun has such a great deal to do with the conditions of the hair, and that is one reason why the hair should never be washed at night. Sometimes shearing is permanently affected by carelessness in this regard. Hair ought never to be "done up" until it is perfectly dried. Wetting the hair to make it smooth is apt to cause injury at the roots.

Many up-to-date hairdressers use the "hot water brush" for drying the hair, declaring its effects to be most satisfactory. The brush is made of metal; the "bristles" are small tubes, containing hot water which is poured into the empty back. The handle is then screwed on, and you have an apparatus that distributes warmth throughout the mass of the hair, quickly drying it.

~**Emma E. Walker M.D.,**
The Pretty Girl Papers (1910)

The purpose of brushing is to polish the little scales that form like shingles on the hair, and to help strengthen the hair muscle.

~Hazel Theresa Gifford,
Fundamentals of Beauty (1944)

The Zander Method of mechanical massage is very effective for reducing flesh. It is simply a vigorous tapping with electrically driven leather-covered hammers. There is a variety of machines comprised in the Zander system for tapping, beating, rubbing, jiggling and exercising almost every part of the body. The fingers of the pianist and the forearms and wrists of the racing automobilist, are made supple by special machines. By

another machine the cushion of flesh on the back of
the neck is beaten down.

~William A. Woodbury,
Beauty Culture (1910)

If you work through the list of measurements and find
that your theoretical answers, derived from the
percentage tables, are hopelessly at variance with the
facts, there is but one answer: you started off with the
wrong figure—you have not the hips that belong to
you and something has got to be done about it. On the
other hand, if your height is three or four inches under
double the girth of your hips, but some of the other
theoretical measurements are radically different from
the facts, you have spotted local imperfections—of
chest, waist, thigh, etc.—and are informed of the
approximate number of inches by which they are
under- or over-developed.

~Sylvia Ullback's Secretary,
Hollywood Undressed, observations of Sylvia as noted to her secretary
(1931)

You Can Have Your Sugar and Diet, Too!
Yes, you're going to be able to include some candy ... or
use sugar every day. ... [D]on't be astonished at this ...
for it isn't as strange as it seems. You, yourself have known

for years that candy before meals takes your appetite away
... just as coffee, before bedtime, helps to keep you awake.

Modern nutritional science has a new term in dieting.
You will hear a great deal about "blood sugar level" in
the next few years ... and nutritionists will certainly
include the use of more sugar in dieting. Now, here it is,
for the first time, in a diet book.

To put it simply, it is this:

1. As you have found out, in previous pages,
   most people get fat because they overeat.
   They eat more calories than their body needs.
2. Why do they overeat? Because they're
   hungry!
3. Why are they hungry? Mainly because
   their "blood sugar level" is low.
4. How can they raise this level quickly?
   Simply by adding sugar to their diet or
   some sweets that contain it.

~Joe Bonomo,
Calorie Counter and Control Guide (1954)

I have a compulsion to take advantage of everything.
When I'm on a plane, for instance, traveling from one
engagement to another, I invariably strap a little
reducing machine to my thighs, my calves, or my

upper arms—whichever section needs to have some fatty tissue broken down.

~Hildegarde,
Over 50—So What! (1963)

If there is any one ingredient that could be called the secret to the Fountain of Youth, I think it has to be water.

I believe in this so strongly that I am developing a "water mask," a kind of rotating sprinkler system that operates on a battery and can be used on your face and body to keep you looking young.

~George Masters,
The Masters Way to Beauty (1977)

No garment has done more to *destroy* the American woman's figure than the combination corset and brassiere one. No one wearing such a garment can attain the correct standing position because of the downward pull of the suspended garters; nor will the wearer ever attain the correct posture. The wearer has no shape, no waistline, flabby, protruding hips, forward shoulders, and will find after wearing the garment for a while that abdominal muscles have sagged thus resulting into constipation and other disorders. Throw this garment away immediately and purchase a step-in girdle.

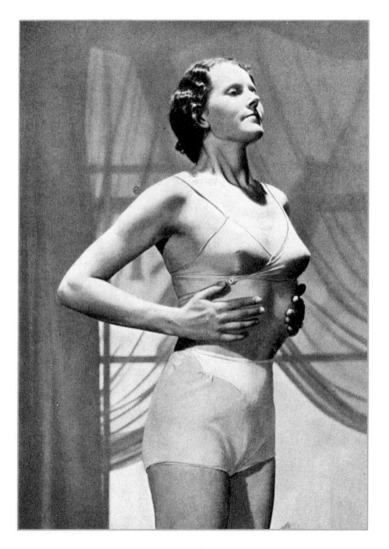

Let us explain this a different way. You will agree that in wearing this garment you wore the front garters short and the back and side garters long. Why did you do this? Because if you didn't wear the back garters long you would never have been able to sit down. Did you ever stop to think what this would do to your figure? Every fat woman has large hips due entirely to the lack of this knowledge. In other words you protrude your hips which naturally give you large hips.

~Lilyan Malmstead,
What Everybody Wants to Know (1928)

> ### *hips = ass*
> In the above quote, and in many books published as recently as even the 1950s, the word "hips" actually means buttocks. There was just no polite way to say it. This gets confusing because "hips" is also used to mean hips.

It is possible to have a brassiere with a kind of pocket into which air can be blown, to improve the shape of the bosom. The *couturiers* make use of them in showing their collections: but, as an innovation for general use, they have provoked a number of protests, as well as smiles.

~Jacqueline Du Pasquier,
A Guide to Elegance (1956)

There lie many great veins, all conducting upward toward the heart. They need to be supported by a stay, or the blood will stagnate in them and not return in proper quantity to the heart. But this is not theory, it is fact, and has been proved again and again. If a tame rabbit is taken and held in an upright position for about half an hour, it becomes unconscious. This is because the blood stagnates in the great veins of the abdomen, and enough does not reach its poor little brain. More interesting however, is a second experiment, in which the animal's abdomen was tightly bandaged. It was then found that standing it upright had not the slightest effect on it. The conclusion that must inevitably be forced on us all is that binding the waist has a distinctly beneficial effect on the circulation of the blood; but this by no means exhausts the advantages we gain from the practise.

~Cora Brown Potter,
The Secrets of Beauty & Mysteries of Health (1908)

Thin lips may be made a bit fuller by the use of this:

Simple Cerate . . . . 10 grams
Essence of Cinnamon . . . . 15 drops
Red Pepper . . . . ½ gram

~William A. Woodbury,
Beauty Culture (1910)

Of course you know that you shouldn't have a permanent when you are not feeling in perfect condition. Don't have one if you have a cold or are menstruating; it would definitely affect the results of the permanent.

~Mildred Graves Ryan and **Velma Phillips,**
Clothes for You (1947)

A correspondent wishes to know what will remove superfluous hair, adding that she is annoyed with such a growth of it on her face that she is the remark of her friends. These unfortunate cases are the result of morbid constitution, freaks of nature which are to be combated as one would eradicate leprosy or scrofula. The extreme growth of hair where it should not be comes from gross living, or is inherited by young persons from those whose

blood was made of too rich materials. Living two or
three generations on overlarded meats, plenty of
pastry, salt meats, ham, and fish, with good old
pickles from brine—in short, what would be called
high living among middle-class people—is pretty
sure to leave its mark on the lips and brow.
Sometimes typhoid fever steps in and arrests the
degeneration by a painful and searching process
which, as it were, burns out the vile particles, and, if
the patients' strength endures, leaves her with an
almost new body. The red, scaly skin peels off, and
leaves a soft, fresh cuticle, pink as a child's; the dry
hair comes out, and a fine, often curling suit
succeeds it, while moles and feminine mustaches
disappear and leave no sign. But this fortunate end
is not secured to order, and there are preferable
ways of renewing the habit of body.

~Mrs. Susan C. D. Power,
The Ugly-Girl Papers (1874)

In this Atomic Age it is an offense to let your face
droop, your muscles sag, and your skin wrinkle.

~Edyth Thornton McLeod,
Lady, Be Lovely (1955)

Here's an infinite wisdom: don't try to improve on the instructions. And that goes for applying home perms, hair tints, face packs, depilatories—any process where chemical action is involved. This is a great female failing . . . a vital upsurge of the creative instinct— misguided!

~Graeme Hall,
Beauty for Girls Who Are Getting On (1970)

Curiouser and Curiouser

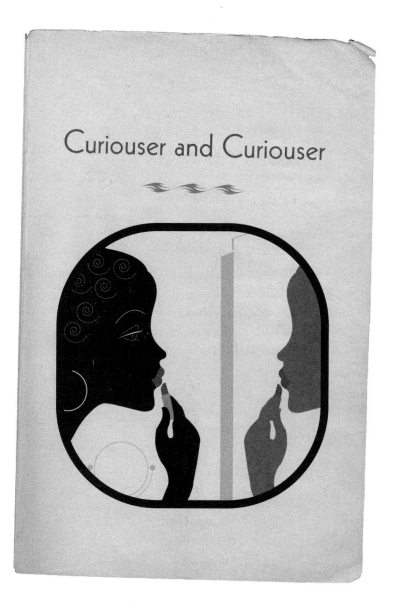

Snacks to serve in your bathroom, makeup for your veins, and a reason to put your pants on backwards. These are beauty tips from beyond, ranging from the merely baffling to the clearly psychotic. I've always firmly believed that everyone deserves one relationship that need only be explained by saying, "It was inexplicable." Now, the same goes for beauty theories, fads, and experiments. This is all the stuff that made me look up from the book, stare into the distance and muse, **hmmm, that's curious**.

Put on a shower cap; grease your face with Vaseline, cold cream or something goopy. Fill the bathroom basin with cold water. Dump in two trays of ice cubes. Using a snorkel (a little rubber tube, one end of which you clamp between your teeth; the other end—open—sticks up out of the water so you can breathe. Any sporting-goods store has these), stick your face down just below the water surface and stay as long as you can. Twenty minutes is ideal. You never saw such skin . . . poreless, glowing.

~Helen Gurley Brown,
The Late Show (1993)

The secrets of "making-up" have hardly all been mentioned, though the list is growing long. What girl does not know that eating lump-sugar wet with Cologne just before going out will make her eyes bright, or that the homelier mode of flirting soap-suds into them has the same effect? Spanish ladies squeeze orange juice into their eyes to make them shine.

~Mrs. Susan C. D. Power,
The Ugly-Girl Papers (1874)

The only harmless means of curling straight hair is to

wet it at night with rectified alcohol, and then to roll it onto soft lead wires.

~The Marquise de Fontenoy,
Eve's Glossary (1897)

Nature has endowed no one with a special skin and muscle flap to prevent that posterior appearance of a valley between two hills. So long as we conform to our present mode of dress, the very shape and fit of any skirt, demand that the wearer do something to prevent that jelly-like quiver and shake, reminiscent of a burlesque performer in action, that travel the abdomen and hips, (also breasts), when their owner is in motion. Clothes cost us much thought, time and money and even a pleated or full gathered skirt reacts to sitting and wind pressures, so why give the appearance of walking out in one's Birthday Clothes and an outer garment, when a "backing" garment is so very comfortable and can be had for such little money?

If one's uncontrolled figure would never encourage approving glances, for pride's sake alone, she should keep it "under cover," and if it is attractive enough to attract applause, its owner should have a sense of security that would make "advertising" unnecessary.

A panty girdle under slacks will not restrict freedom of motion. If statistics were available to show the percentage of our gruesome sex crimes attributable to the uncontrolled female form on parade, doubtless it would prove most startling.

~Mary Jane Moore, R.N.,
You Can Too! (1950)

Asslessness

Let's put Nurse Moore's last remark aside for a moment, shocking though it may be. Hope you got that she actually finds the fact that women have an ass to be offensive. The "flap of skin" she mentions seems to her to be the ideal.

The note *hips = ass* from the last chapter may also be of some help to you here.

Yeah, and the sex crimes remark? Really uncalled for.

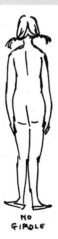

NO
GIRDLE

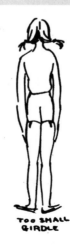

TOO SMALL
GIRDLE

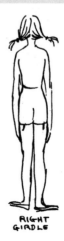

RIGHT
GIRDLE

Now that you have created a secret spa and conjured up some secret recipes, why not share your secrets? I'm not recommending you have a block party in your bathroom, but it can be a lovely thing to invite the man in your life to share your beautiful bath.

If the mood is tender, your bath is an unrivaled place for soft conversation. You can exchange ideas and back rubs at the same time. Serve cool wine or favorite drinks along with elegant canapés.

Keep a jar of macadamia nuts in the medicine cabinet and if the "double dip" is spontaneous surprise him with their hiding place and eat them right out of the jar accompanied by a pitcher of martinis.

~Alexandra York,
Back to Basics Natural Beauty Handbook (1977)

The *patch*, as it first came in, was one of the most harmless and effective aids to beauty ever invented. It was but a tiny, mole-like spot of black velvet or silk, which was used to draw attention to some particular feature, as well as to enhance, by contrast, the fairness of the cheek. Thus, if a girl was conscious of a pretty dimple on her chin, or of long eyebrows; if her forehead formed the best part of her face, or her mouth — she cunningly placed the little patch near it, and consequently every time you looked at her your eye was insensibly drawn by the patch to the best feature, so that you partly forget any less handsome detail. To an accustomed eye, the patch gives a singular finish to the toilet; it is like the seal on a letter or the frame to a picture. You see the grey powdered curls and the bright eyes, and the low, luxurious bodice, and the ribbon necklet around the throat — and if the patch is absent, it is instantly missed, and the whole toilet seems incomplete. This crafty little piece of vanity was afterwards vulgarized, of course. . . . [T]he tiny round spot was transformed into a star or crescent, that increased in size and multiplied in number — blind vanity forgot that in trying to draw attention to all her features at once, she drew attention to none; and, later on, it ran into such absurd extremes that ships, chariots, and horses, and other devices in black paper, began to disfigure the female visage, and at last the whole face was bespatted with vulgar shapes, having no meaning, unless sometimes a political one, and being of no value to beauty whatever.

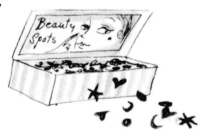

~Mrs. H. R. Haweis,
The Art of Beauty (1878)

Bleu Vegetal

Venetian chalk	5 ounces
Methylene blue	3½ drachms
Gum acacia	2 drachms

Mix the powders with sufficient water to form a mass that can be rolled into sticks. This is used to mark blue veins which a coating of balm or paints has concealed. It requires some dexterity to apply it in a natural manner. Breathe upon one of the sticks and rub it on the inside of a white glove, then trace the vein with the kid. It could be done more deftly with a Japanese paint brush.

~Ella Adelia Fletcher,
The Woman Beautiful (1901)

Here is the big secret: take your foundation to bed for ten minutes. The move does more than refresh your bones. What happens in this—the epidermis, or outer layer of skin, absorbs the foundation, causing a slight expansion of the skin and subsequently a temporary disappearance of tiny lines and wrinkles. For a long-lasting finish, apply a second coat upon arising.

~John Robert Powers and **Mary Sue Miller,**
Secrets of Charm (1954)

Everyone absorbs makeup through their skin, but some people absorb it much faster than others. I call this the "disappearing makeup." I have a friend who swears that before she is ready to go out of her house in the morning, her makeup has disappeared. This happened to some people often and to others only at certain times: during menstruation, during times of stress, when particularly tired, or when dieting.

~**Victoria Principal,**
The Beauty Principal (1984)

If you have the least suspicion of a curl in your hair, brushing *around* rather than *straight* will bring it out.

~**Florence Courtenay,**
Physical Beauty (1922)

How to Cure Constipation

EXERCISE 1	Position:	Lying on back, hands under small of back.
		(a) Cross ankles and bend knees bringing them up quickly over abdomen.
MUSIC: Ballet No. 2, Part I		(b) Extend them forcibly back to floor in same direction
Standard Classic Ballet Bar		you came up in. (See Figure No. 13.)
EXERCISE 2	Position:	Lying with trunk on table face downward, arms extended straight above, grasping either side of table.
		Raise legs up to level of table. Keep knees and toes rigid and extended.
MUSIC: "Burgundy"		(Try not to do this exercise with back muscles. Hands are
(See Figure No. 12.)		there for support only.)
EXERCISE 3	Position:	Lying on back, hands under small of back.
		Bend knees, feet resting on floor, crossing ankles, bring knees over abdomen, then stretch out knees in direc-

---

HOW TO CURE CONSTIPATION

MUSIC: "Weiner Waltz"		tion of left side and continue forward over to right side, beginning to bend knees as they approach abdomen. After rotating for 8 times change and go in opposite directions.
EXERCISE 4	Position:	Lying on left side, on left arm, both legs straight, the right over the left, and together. Bring both knees up to abdomen and force back to position quickly.
MUSIC: "The Glow-Worm"		Change to other side.

EXERCISE 5   Position :   Lying on back, hands behind neck.

(a) Bend knees over abdomen.
(b) Drop knees to right.
(c) Sway knees over to left side.
(d) Bring knees over abdomen and continue rocking back and forth. At the same time, breathe deeply with the abdominal cavity.

MUSIC: "Spring, Beautiful Spring"

The best way to polish or to complete the polishing of nails is to bend the fingers on to the palm of the hand by bending the knuckles and first joint while keeping the last joint straight, and to rub briskly the nails on the palm of your other hand. This not only polishes the nails, but also massages the skin at the root, so that the blood supply of the nails is improved and the growth of the nail is strengthened; then they become smoother, with an absence of ribs and ridges, provided always that the skin at the root is not undermined.

~Cora Brown Potter,
The Secrets of Beauty and Mysteries of Health (1908)

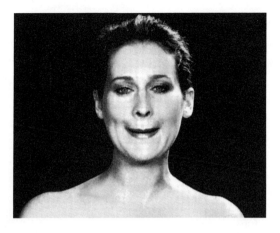

A very ancient and wonderful French manual, written some time during the seventeenth century, asserts that linen bed sheets are pernicious to beauty, and recommends most urgently the use of chamois leather ones. Now, chamois leather has been used for many purposes, from a shoe to a card-case, but it is only lately that it has been once more called into requisition for sheets. The idea originated with a lady whose skin was of marvelous delicacy, and who had made a careful study of the book in question. Chamois leather sheets are now becoming quite popular, and women who use them travel about carrying with them their own sheets, smartly trimmed with colored ribbons.

~The Marquise de Fontenoy,
Eve's Glossary (1897)

Try taking 250 mg. of niacin before a special evening out (I always do this before an important shoot) to make your eyes sparkle and your skin glow.

~Beverly Johnson,
True Beauty (1994)

The Niacin Flush

Niacin is an important B vitamin that is sometimes prescribed for lowering cholesterol. Taking niacin supplements often produces extreme redness of the face and other parts of the body along with a sensation of uncontrollable heat and itching. This "niacin flush" is considered by some (although clearly not all) to be an unpleasant side effect. In fact, time released supplements are now made to prevent it. The flush is ultimately harmless, though, and is the result of vasodilatation and an increase in histamines—similar to the way your body reacts to an insect bite.

I have to shop with great care and use ingenuity. There's usually a label in the pants that says "Front." I turn that around and get in backward. The front, which is supposed to be flat for the stomach, works perfectly for my flat behind. The back part, which is roomier, fits perfectly over the part where I'm supposed to be flat but am not. It's marvelous how

things can work for you if you're willing to try
something a little different.

~Polly Bergen,
Polly's Principles (1974)

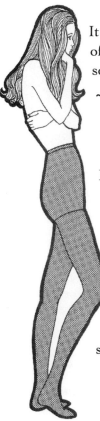

It is a mistake to suppose that hair piled on top
of the head can add to apparent height. To do
so, only puts the eyes in the wrong position.

~Francis Mary Steele and **Elizabeth Livingston Steele
Adams,**
Beauty of Form and Grace of Vesture (1892)

Four pairs of stockings in a neutral skin color
keep you in stockings at all times. When one
runs, buy another. Buy your hose in the same
color. When one leg of your pantyhose runs,
cut it off and save the top of the good leg.
You can wear two one-legged pantyhose at
the same time, since the panties are thin
enough to be comfortable when worn
together. If you have two "partials" of the
same leg, turn one leg inside out.

~Carole Jackson,
Color Me Beautiful (1980)

Holiday Wear: You can now buy disposable panties and nightwear. These save washing and leave space in your suitcase for souvenirs.

~Margaret Cullen,
Good Grooming and Clothes Care (1971)

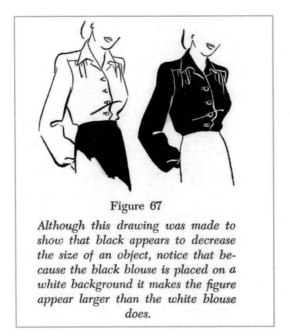

Figure 67

Although this drawing was made to show that black appears to decrease the size of an object, notice that because the black blouse is placed on a white background it makes the figure appear larger than the white blouse does.

Now for a surprise! You can reduce your breasts. I have an absolute, sure way. But wait until warm weather.

You'll feel much better if you do it then. You must rely entirely upon a special diet. . . . For three days in succession do this. When you get up in the morning, drink a glass of hot or cold water. Two hours after your water, drink six ounces of buttermilk. Two hours later, drink another six ounces. Do this every two hours until bed-time. Remember this must be done three days in succession. . . . This buttermilk diet never fails.

~Sylvia of Hollywood,
No More Alibis (1934)

A simple and pleasant way to exercise the muscles connected with the bosom is to bend from the waist while you are brushing your hair, and brush rhythmically with a brush in each hand.

~Robert Alan Franklyn, M.D.,
Developing Bosom Beauty (1959)

Go after that fagged-out feeling with a bristled brush, and while you are restoring your normal spirits you are giving your scalp worthwhile attention and taking care of your chinline, too. Women are frankly bored with hairbrush theories, yet when you are tired, "headachey," and discouraged, first comb the hair away from the face, and then use a stiff brush from the temples to the crown, and from behind the ears to the center, and from the nape of the head to the top of it. To save time, a pair of brushes can be used, working from both temples at once.

~How to Attain and Retain Beauty (1935)
from The Home Library of Great Britain

There are garments, as there are faces and natures, which have no "bar" in them—nothing which stops with sudden shock your pleasure in them, nothing that dissatisfies or perplexes you.

~Mrs. H. R. Haweis,
The Art of Beauty (1878)

That Sounds Dirty

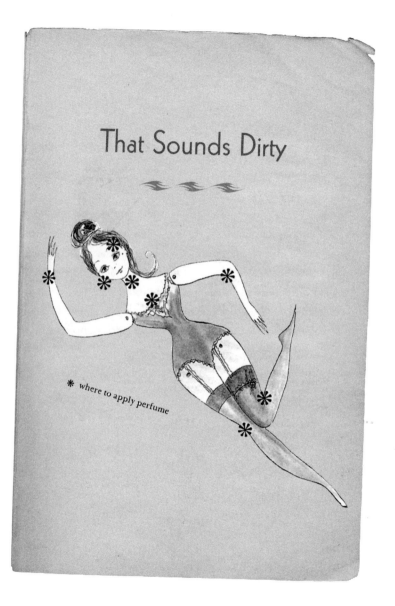

* where to apply perfume

Clandestine rituals, compromised elegance, and double-entendres. Visit a country of pantyless women, learn the ancient history of nipple glitter, and read a quote about baby oil that you'll want to have professionally steam-cleaned from your brain. Some of these tips are pornographic by pure accident, others are tips for your most intimate areas and occasions. Face it: If you spend as much time rubbing yourself down as these women do, people will talk.

There have been exaggerated claims for breast massage and the practice has been abused to a considerable degree. Especially is this true when it is practiced by people who are uninformed or untrained.

~Joe Bonomo,
Reduce and Beautify Your Figure (1954)

Some time ago twin lipsticks made their appearance, both in the same color. One gave the lips a shiny glitter, while the other left a dull luster. The first was called Hussy and the other Lady. Ladies bought Hussy so fast and frequently that it outsold Lady many times. (I never did hear whether hussies bought Lady or not.) We might as well admit there's a dash of hussy in all ladies. Some corner of your personality must have its opportunity to flaunt a hussy mood now and then: lipstick or what have you.

~Ruth Harper Larison,
Those Enduring Young Charms (1942)

This description is for a massage, while lying on the floor with the feet elevated on the back of an upturned kitchen type chair, which will offer foot and leg elevation of about 45 degrees. . . . Place the chair on its front, with the top cross-piece of the back and the front of the seat touching the floor and the legs in the air. . . . Place nude self on your back with feet elevated as above described and use cover for parts of the body not being massaged.

~**Mary Jane Moore, R.N.,**
You Can Too! (1950)

I want to help you master the secrets of nighttime makeup. I want your face to shine with the confidence and beauty that reflects your own personal fashion statement. Maybe your statement will be Mystery. Or Exotica. Or Sensuality. Or Allure. Or simply Good Time.

~**Sandy Linter,**
Disco Beauty (1979)

For developing the breasts there is only one course which may possibly succeed. Take up swimming and singing, with an instructor for both.

~Sylvia Ullback's Secretary,
Hollywood Undressed, observations of Sylvia as noted to her secretary (1931)

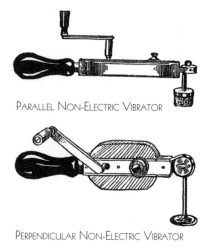

PARALLEL NON-ELECTRIC VIBRATOR

PERPENDICULAR NON-ELECTRIC VIBRATOR

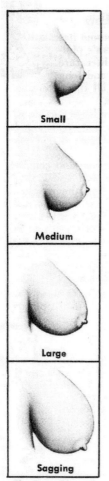

The Four General Types Of Breasts

(from top to bottom: Small, Medium, Large, Sagging)

Egyptian beauties were the first to use body glitter, gilding their nipples with an elegant gold frost. When you are entertaining a special someone, you might try using a gold or bronze mica powder on this super-sexy part of you, for a special under-negligee surprise.

~**Barbara Walden,**
Easy Glamour (1981)

Johnson & Johnson Baby Oil
That was some trip, that was — your mother oiling you and patting you all over with scented oil. The comforting sensation is still with you, isn't it? Get acquainted with it again: buy yourself a big bottle of baby oil, and keep it on your bathroom shelf.

~**Stan Place,**
Stan Place's Guide to Makeup (1981)

The shape, size, firmness and erectness of the breast, also their relation to the size and contour of the body are all taken into account when a woman is appraised for her charm. By strengthening the supporting muscles, exercise can cause the breasts to be held more erectly and carried more proudly, thus greatly enhancing the entire personality.

~**Ern** and **Bud Westmore,**
Beauty, Glamour and
Personality (1947)

Hips may be reduced by hitting them smartly on the floor. As you lie back with your knees bent, roll from side to side thumping the hips each time against the floor.

~**Mildred Graves Ryan**
and **Velma Phillips,**
Clothes for You (1947)

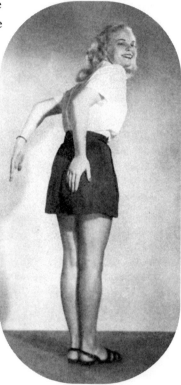

Give yourself a daily spanking to reduce those fleshy spots on your hips, thighs, calves, and arms.

The beauty machines are changing our lives.

These days, when the phone rings, you don't say, "Hang on while I turn off the vacuum cleaner." Instead it's more likely to be, "Wait t-t-till I t-t-turn off my v-v-vibrator!"

. . . It's a little bit like having your own beauty club at home. When I was growing up, my daydreams of luxury living were a combination of princess and movie star. I could visualize myself in a pink satin setting with my gorgeous husband—and, in the background, a resident hairdresser, cosmetologist, masseuse, and dietician, all hanging around for Madame to snap her fingers (or whistle).

Wouldn't that have been great? *Quick, Mario—my massage!*

. . . As a busy woman with a seventy-four hour day, you've probably had the same daydream. Before we join hands in mourning for the loss of this dream, let me point out that the dream isn't really lost. It has come true, but on modern terms. . . .

There's a belt massager which makes me feel like an old-style shimmy dancer. *Quick, Mario—my tango records!* It shakes all the kinks out while exercising and firming flabby hips and thighs.

~Eve Nelson,
Take It From Eve (1968)

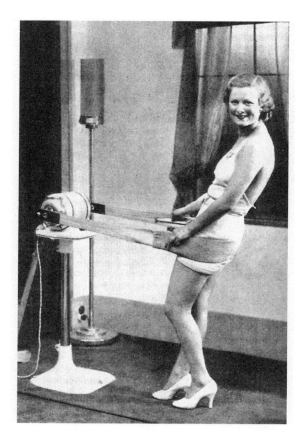

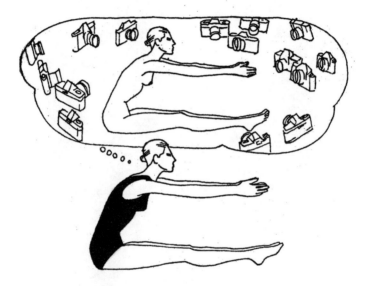

Crucial to your total look of beauty is body control. If you don't have it, start working on it instantly. You can begin this very second and here's how: *Pretend you're naked with forty cameras shooting you from all angles.* This is a trick I learned from Natasha Lytess, who was Marilyn Monroe's drama, diction, and body-control coach. . . . Marilyn Monroe's super body control didn't come naturally. She was rigorously trained by Natasha, so well trained that the control looked natural.

Anyone can do it. You start by pretending that you're naked with forty imaginary cameras shooting you from every possible angle—up, down, front, back, sideways—on your cheekbones, chinbone, nose, neckline, shoulderline, hipline, bosoms, stomach, thighs, arms and legs, all over, anywhere and everywhere. . . . It's a trick you can practice anywhere, even out in public. Maybe you have a secret yen to be a streaker. Here's your chance. Pretend you're nude with the cameraman chasing you. (Be sure you're only pretending or it could be the cops.) . . . You might need to pin notes in a few strategic spots in your house to jog your memory: *I'm naked with the cameras shooting.*

~George Masters,
The Masters Way to Beauty (1977)

Be glad you don't live in Czechoslovakia or the Soviet Union. On October 22, 1969, newspapers reported a shortage of panties in Prague. Cause: a lack of equipment, labor shortage, and no funds to buy materials such as elastic. The nation teetered nervously on the brink of a women's riot. One woman was quoted saying, "When shall we be able to dress from the bottom up instead of from the top down? I have been walking around without panties for a month!"

~Lolita R. Linzano,
The Wonderful New World of Women (1976)

Choose a color and make it your trademark. Yellow has always been a happy color for me, and I wear a lot of it. (Once actor Johnny Forsythe saw me wearing my bright yellow angora sweater in a gift shop and commented, "Barbara, you look just like a delicious yellow ice cream cone." I loved looking "delicious"!) You may want to make one color the theme of your wardrobe.

~Barbara Walden,
Easy Glamour (1981)

What grandma may have been too reticent to tell you is that we should brush our pubic hair. This should be done with a small round brush of its own. Brush only the front part, gently upward, so it remains shiny, curly, and crisp—a fitting wreath around a whirlpool of joy. Don't forget to give this outside hair the care it deserves, shampooing it weekly with a good, mild shampoo—it is hair, isn't it? I have heard from a very reputable hair expert in Paris that pubic hair when brushed and taken care of, won't keep falling out. Who wants to have a bald head—anywhere?

~Stella Jones Reichman,
Great Big Beautiful Doll (1977)

These don't just SOUND dirty.

Please Come To Our Little Den of Iniquity:

If you're invited for a group swing, don't immediately reach for your petticoats and your square-dancing skirt. Nowadays such events rarely have a caller, and your petticoats would be sure to get in the way (not to mention the laced bodice!). . . . Since this book should serve as a dressing guide to the modern women in all likely (and unlikely) circumstances, I'd like to pass on a few pointers:

Number 1.

Don't wear anything that binds or leaves marks on the body. It's very unattractive.

Number 2.

Omit stockings and underwear, if possible. Not only do they leave marks on the body when they come off—they're also likely to get in your way and be unnecessarily cumbersome.

Number 3.

Wear sexy clothes. They should be very body conscious (like the guests) and should emphasize your best features. Whatever clings is fine. This is a perfect occasion to wear any see-through garments you own, though even in this situation the see-through blouse should not merely be a soft windowpane, but should rather be suggestive. If everything's laid out for inspection, some people will stay with the window shopping and never come in.

Number 4.

Sew name tags on all articles of personal property—it's easier to reclaim then afterward.

~Polly Bergen,
I'd Love to But What'll I Wear (1977)

The only possible colour for the court is white. For players of both sexes, shorts are suitable; but many women still prefer to wear a little skirt, with a sleeveless blouse or perfectly laundered polo shirt in linen or poplin. Too delicate a material is easily ruined by perspiration. (It is essential to shave under the arms.)

You shirt should be very long, or attached to a pair of briefs—or to your shorts, all in one piece; if not, your arm movements, in serving, may pull it loose from the belt, and there goes your claim to elegance!

~Jacqueline Du Pasquier,
A Guide to Elegance (1956)

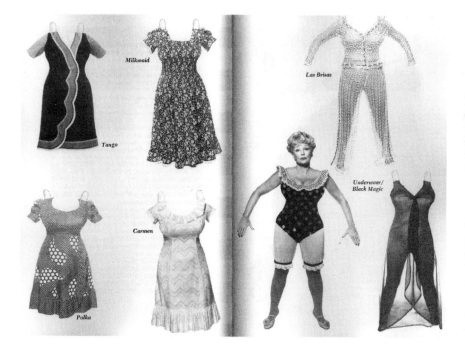

Tango

Milkmaid

Las Brisas

Polka

Carmen

Underwear/
Black Magic

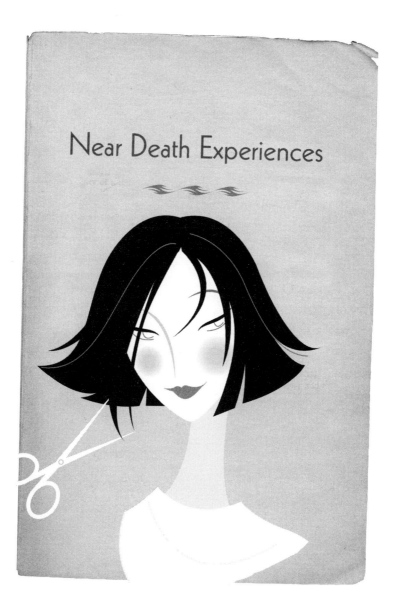

Near Death Experiences

Gasoline shampoo, radioactive mud baths, and early attempts at electrolysis gone terribly, terribly wrong. Sometimes there is a fine line between personal improvement and attempted suicide. Among the health and beauty aids featured here you'll find asbestos, mercury, lead, arsenic, and opium. In most cases, these girls have no idea that their plans are flawed and a minor mistake can mean death or disfigurement. Dangerous and stupid? Why, yes, but do keep in mind how modern indulgences like Botox, tanning beds, and bootleg ephedra will look through the lens of time. Oh, wait. Those already look bad.

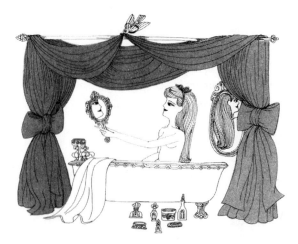

A sulphur bath requires a shallow pan of coals with a tin water-pan above it, and an elevated seat over the whole. Sulphur is thrown on the coals, which mingles with the steam, and enters the system by the pores, which are opened by the vapor. The patient, brazier, and chair must be enveloped with a waterproof covering in the closest manner, leaving only the head exposed, so that no sulphurous vapor can possibly be breathed, as that would be suffocation at once.

~Mrs. Susan C. D. Power,
The Ugly-Girl Papers (1874)

Parisians have recently been washing their hair in gasoline. Not because they believe it will cause hair to grow, but for the same purpose that it is used upon a spotted garment—to cleanse the garment and remove the spots. Also gasoline makes the hair soft and silken of texture. . . .

I myself have used gasoline a few times on my hair, but always try to keep it away from the scalp as much as possible. I cannot believe that gasoline is good for the scalp. I take the gasoline shampoo somewhat as I do the water bath for the hair. I wash it in a bowl of gasoline, pour the first bowlful and wash it through another, then another, until the last bowlful is entirely clean. Let as little gasoline as possible get to the scalp. But the shampoo is always taken on the morning of a clear day. Never do I have it done while there is a light or fire in the room. If I did, there would be no more Lina Cavalieri.

~Lina Cavalieri,
My Secrets of Beauty (1914)

One serious objection against all false hair is that it is a disease carrier. If you wear it, treat it as you would your own hair. Brush it often, clean it in gasoline (this, of course, you do not do to your own hair) and dry it in the sun and open air.

~Florence Courtenay,
Physical Beauty (1922)

Complexion Improvers: Most of the preparations sold under this or similar names contain corrosive sublimate, perchloride of mercury. This powerful drug must be used with caution, as it produces marked alteration in, and hardening of, the skin. On account of its strong germicidal properties it has long been used by surgeons for cleansing their hands for operations, but too often has its action been so severe as to cause the hands to become very rough and the skin so cracked and painful as even to necessitate them giving up work for weeks.

No preparations containing mercury should be allowed to come into contact with any rings or other ornaments, as it corrodes the metal and loosens the setting of the stones.

It often happens that their use for toilet purposes is profitable to the seller, because, their nature being unknown to the buyer, one or more other preparations must be purchased from the same source to remove the ill effects of the first.

We can, fortunately, minimize or entirely remove the undesirable action of this drug by adding a little yolk of egg to the lotion as:

(1) Corrosive Sublimate 1 gr., Camphor 2 gr., Zinc Sulphate 5 gr., Rectified Spirit 30 drops, Yolk of Egg 1 dr./ Rose Water to 1 oz.

~Cora Brown Potter,
The Secrets of Beauty and Mysteries of Health (1908)

A certain preparation advertised to produce rosy cheeks without the help of rouge consists of a powdered silicious sponge. Examined under the microscope, the preparation is seen to be made up of multitudes of tiny, silicious needles.

These sharp spines stick into the skin, irritating it, thus causing it to redden.

~**Emma E. Walker. M.D.,**
The Pretty Girl Papers (1910)

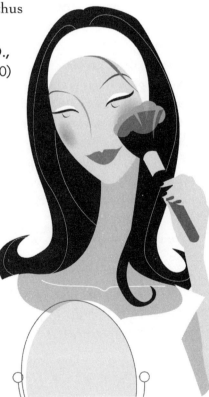

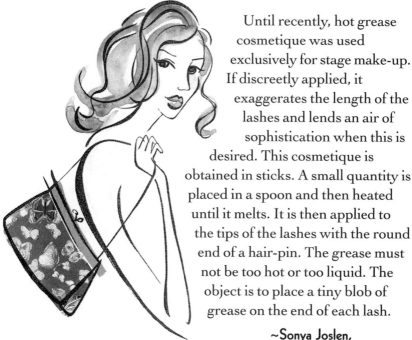

Until recently, hot grease cosmetique was used exclusively for stage make-up. If discreetly applied, it exaggerates the length of the lashes and lends an air of sophistication when this is desired. This cosmetique is obtained in sticks. A small quantity is placed in a spoon and then heated until it melts. It is then applied to the tips of the lashes with the round end of a hair-pin. The grease must not be too hot or too liquid. The object is to place a tiny blob of grease on the end of each lash.

~Sonya Joslen,
The Way to Beauty (1937)

A girl who spent her vacation last August in the hills of Connecticut told me how she managed her bathing without a bath-room.

We have those luxuries all the year, and it is fun to go without them in vacation. I take a two-quart pail with me, so that I can always have hot water any time and anywhere within a few minutes. The best alcohol lamp I have ever used cost me just twelve cents. It is made in the form of a metal cup filled with asbestos; over the top is fitted a piece of wire netting. I buy a pint of wood alcohol which costs, as a rule, twenty cents. Two tablespoonfuls of the alcohol will thoroughly wet the asbestos, and will boil two quarts of water. . . .

In England, even when there are bath-rooms in the house, it is a very common custom to have what is called a tray or sponge bath in the dressing-room. This is made of tin, is four or five feet in diameter, and has a shallow rim. It is like a bread pan, only much larger. . . . The so-called tray may be partly filled with water, the sponge dipped into it and squeezed out over the body, or one may step into the tray and use water from a basin down one side. The tray is large enough to sit down in. If you are unable to find such a tub, it can easily be made by an ordinary tinsmith.

~Emma E. Walker, M.D.,
The Pretty Girl Papers (1910)

TO REMOVE AND PREVENT WRINKLES
There is a curious recipe called *Aura and Cephalus* which is of Grecian origin, as its name would indicate, and is said to have been most efficacious in removing and preventing wrinkles from the faces of Athenian ladies.

Put some powder of the best myrrh upon an iron plate, sufficiently heated to melt the gum gently, and when it liquefies, cover your head with a napkin, and hold your face over the myrrh at a proper distance to receive the fumes without inconvenience. I will observe, however, that if this experiment produces any symptoms of headache, it better be discontinued at once.

~Lola Montez,
The Arts and Secrets of Beauty (1854)

Lola Montez seduced royalty, inspired poems and paintings, drove men to deadly duels, and carried a riding whip with her wherever she went.

In her autobiography, Lola writes, "To be beautiful! What power and what good fortune! To need only to appear in order to attract all eyes to oneself, to exact homage, to inspire love and enthusiasm!"

My favorite Lola story is about the day she met King Ludwig I of Bavaria. He was immediately taken with her beauty, and foolishly insisted that her perfect form must surely be the result of some complicated foundation garment. Lola grabbed a pair of nearby scissors and sliced open the bodice of her dress. Of course, this only deepened the king's infatuation. Some say their affair led indirectly to the revolution of 1848.

Lola died of consumption at the age of 41. She was penniless. She is buried in Brooklyn, N.Y.

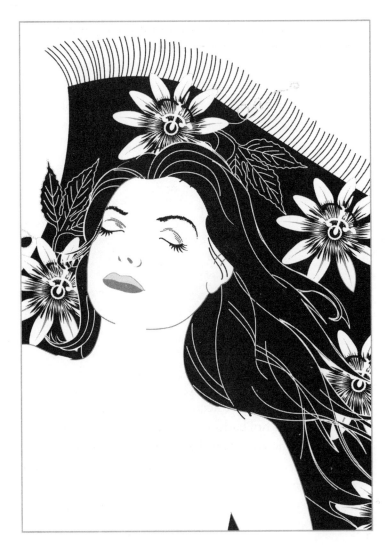

The opium found in the stalks of flowering lettuce refines the skin singularly, and may be used clear, instead of the soap which sells so high. Rub the milky juice collected from broken stems of coarse garden lettuce over the face at night, and wash with a solution of ammonia in the morning.

~Mrs. Susan C. D. Power,
The Ugly-Girl Papers (1874)

Aside from the parching effect which white lotions containing lead or bismuth invariably have on the skin, there is another far more disfiguring. . . . This will occur where gas is escaping from the pipes or furnace, or when sulphurous fumes of any description are encountered. An instance once came under the writer's observation, which proved a lesson to all to whom the facts were known.

The belle of a gay party at a mineral-spring resort was envied of all for her lovely complexion, which she positively asserted was wholly natural; and indeed, one could not detect any artificial aid to its purity. Concluding to try one of the hot baths of the establishment, she was informed by the attendant that it would be best for her, if she used any cosmetic, to thoroughly wash her face before going into the bath-room. It would never do to follow this advice, since such a course would be a tacit admission of what she had strenuously denied. So, with a highly indignant manner at the suspicion conveyed in the warning, our belle ignored the latter and proceeded to the bath. Her attendant silently performed her duties, and at the end of fifteen or twenty minutes left her charge in order that the latter might dress herself. Suddenly there was a sound of sorrow from the little room, and our belle rushed frantically forth, with her face and neck about the color of those of a dingy mulatto. The fumes of the sulphurous water had changed the color of the cosmetic which she did use on her face, and the poor girl was disconsolate, and obliged to seclude herself. No one had the heart to ask her again if she did not use some complexion lotion, for she was doubly punished.

~The Butterick Publishing Company,
Beauty: Its Attainment and Preservation (1890)

The mention of arsenic naturally brings me to those drugs which specially act on the skin and complexion. In the East antimony and arsenic have long been used for this purpose.

Their original prescription yet remains. . . . It is a remedy which has stood the test of time and the recent advances of science.

The prescription of this ancient beautifier is 1-100 of a grain of arsenic and two grains of black pepper. One of these pills should be taken after dinner. It clears the complexion and brings a ruddy glow to the lips and cheeks, but it should only be taken when the tongue is uncoated by fur on rising in the morning, and never if there is any tendency to redness or roughness of the skin, or by those who suffer from flatulence.

~Cora Brown Potter,
The Secrets of Beauty and Mysteries of Health (1908)

The dark circles under the eyes are usually caused by an impairment of the chemical constitution of the blood or an impoverishment of the system by prolonged study, lack of sleep, or dissipation of any kind. External treatment is sometimes effective, but not permanent while the cause exists. Bathe frequently with cold water and use friction. A little turpentine liniment may be rubbed into the skin daily, or weak ammonia — one part to four parts water — care being taken to let neither get into the eyes.

~William A. Woodbury,
Beauty Culture (1910)

Mercurial lotion, which may not be used if there is any eruption of the face, is the strongest bleach made and is to be brought into requisition with great discrimination, I think. It is made by dissolving ten grains of corrosive sublimate crystals in half a pint each of rose and distilled water. The work should be done by a chemist.

~**Margaret Mixter,**
Health and Beauty Hints (1910)

Let no one persuade you to have melted paraffin injected under your skin to fill out hollows in your cheeks or to model your nose on more Grecian lines. The paraffin, some warm day, will melt down in little tears, giving your face an odd bumpy look not to be got rid of except by operations to remove the paraffin from the tissues.

~**Dorothy Cocks,**
The Etiquette of Beauty (1927)

Cigarette smoking—now a firmly established custom amongst Englishwomen—tends to blacken the teeth. This blackening, though very unsightly, does not injure the teeth in any way—indeed, the deposit seems to exercise a preservative action upon them.

~**Stanley H. Redgrove,**
The Cream of Beauty (1931)

Mud or clay masks suit the greasy skin. In this country the best and most popular form of mud is fuller's earth, which comes from Reigate. Radioactive packs are made from mud taken from the river St. Gellert.

~Sonya Joslen,
The Way to Beauty (1937)

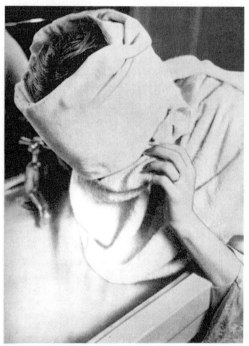

ARRANGEMENT OF TOWELS BEFORE TREATMENT FOR
BLACKHEADS ON CHIN

It sometimes happens that feminine beauty is a little marred by an unfeminine growth of hair on the upper lip, or on the neck and arms, and sometimes the shin. I have known several unfortunate ladies to produce ulcers and dangerous sores by compounds which they used for the purpose of removing these blemishes. Caustic preparations of lime, arsenic, and potash have been used for this purpose with the above results.

~Madame Lola Montez,
The Arts and Secrets of Beauty (1853)

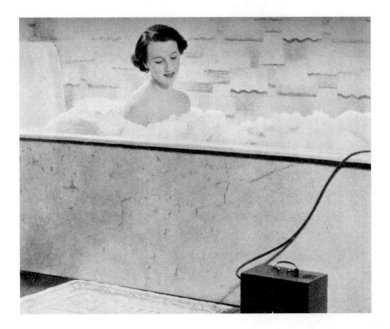

One of the first principles of these home remedies for the ears is to keep these organs free of wax. . . . This treatment must be carefully administered, so the delicate structure will not be injured. A safe way of removing the wax is with a wire hairpin.

~Margaret Mixter,
Health and Beauty Hints (1910)

The following lotion may be used three times a week, or less often, for checking excessive underarm perspiration after the parts have been bathed with salt water and dried: Mix one-half ounce of formaldehyde with one pint water and apply to armpits.

~Lois Leeds,
Beauty and Health (1927)

I have recently seen many women who had undergone X-ray treatment to have the hair removed from their upper lips. The hair was gone, to be sure, but the center of the lip had a curious dead look. . . .

The other method for removing superfluous hair (is) still something of a curiosity. It is a punching procedure, by means of a hollow cylinder, which resembles an old fashioned watch-key with a sharpened end. These cylinders are attached to rotating tubes, something like a dentist's apparatus. When such a machine is put in motion, by electricity, the cylinder rotates around its axis with great velocity. One grasps the handle of the tube, places it on the hair which is to be removed, and presses it vigorously into the skin. The hair, together with its root, is separated from the surrounding tissue and can now be pulled out. This method, which can be learned easily, is almost painless (the skin may be anaesthetized with ethyl chloride) and from 250 to 300 hairs can be removed at one sitting. But it has the disadvantage, to put it mildly, that large parts of the tissue is removed too.

~Helena Rubinstein,
The Art of Feminine Beauty (1930)

Occasional douching seems desirable in the interests of cleanliness and hygiene.

An extremely pleasant, highly antiseptic, perfumed toilet water for use for the purposes under consideration can be made as follows . . .

Antiseptic and Perfumes Toilet Water
Formaldehyde solution, B. P 20
Rose-water, undiluted . . . . to 100
Patchouli oil . . . . a trace

Formaldehyde itself is a gas, and is sold in the form of an aqueous solution often described as "40 per cent." though it is frequently a little weaker than this. The solution is one of the most powerful germicides known to science but, as it is very irritating, it must be well diluted before use.

~Stanley H. Redgrove,
The Cream of Beauty (1931)

The fairest skins belong to people in the earliest stage of consumption, or those of a scrofulous nature. This miraculous clearness and brilliance is due to the constant purgation which wastes the consumptive, or to the issue which relieves the system of impurities by one outlet. We must secure purity of the blood by less exhaustive methods.

~Mrs. Susan C. D. Power,
The Ugly-Girl Papers (1874)

More and more women realize that many of the things they formerly had done at beauty shops can be done at home. This is true. There are many things you can do at home, as well as some things you should not try to do.

~Hazel Theresa Gifford,
Fundamentals of Beauty (1944)

Get all cleaned up. Get healthy. Get your spine straight. Then sit down and write your own book.

~Elizabeth Hawes,
Good Grooming (1942)

Acknowledgments:

Many thanks to Jory Adam, Deborah Ager,
Bill Beverly, Talia Cohen, Jennifer Coia, Alexis
Cuadrado, Laura Dail, Maria Elias, Molly and Caitlin
FitzSimons, Nate Knaebel, Geri Kym, Tina Pohlman,
the New York Pubic Library, and my family.

Excerpt from *The Natural Way to Super Beauty* by
Mary Ann Crenshaw. Published by Dell Publishing
Company. Copyright 1974 by Mary Ann Crenshaw.
Used by permission of the author.

Excerpt from *Always Ask a Man* by Arlene Dahl.
Published by Prentice-Hall. Copyright 1965 by
Arlene Dahl. Used by permission of the author.

Excerpt from *The Beautiful Woman* by Rita Gam.
Published by Prentice-Hall. Copyright 1967 by Rita
Gam. Used by permission of the author.

Excerpt from *True Beauty* by Beverly Johnson.
Published by Warnerbooks. Copyright 1994 by
Beverly Johnson. Used by permission of the author.

Excerpt from *A Year of Beauty and Health* by Beverly
and Vidal Sassoon. Copyright 1975 by Beverly and
Vidal Sassoon. Used by permission of the authors.